The 14 Day Rule and Huma Embryo Research

This assessment of Britain's influential 14 day rule governing embryo research explores how and why it became the *de facto* global standard for research into human fertilisation and embryology, arguing that its influence and stability offers valuable lessons for successful biological translation.

One of the most important features of the 14 day rule, the authors claim, is its reliance on sociological as well as ethical, legislative, regulatory and scientific principles. The careful integration of social expectations and perceptions, as well as sociological definitions of the law and morality, into the development of a robust legislative infrastructure of 'human fertilisation and embryology', enabled what has come to be known as the Warnock Consensus – a solid and enduring public acceptance that has enabled successive parliamentary approval for controversial areas of scientific research in the UK, such as stem cell research and mitochondrial donation, for over 30 years. These important sociological insights are increasingly relevant to new biotranslational challenges such as human germline gene editing and the use of AI assisted technologies in human reproduction. As the legislation around the 14 day rule begins to be reviewed worldwide, the important lessons we can learn from its global and enduring significance will apply not only to future legislation governing embryo research, but to the future of biological translation more widely.

An important volume for those interested in reproductive studies, biogovernance and biological translation, it is suitable for researchers, clinicians and students in medicine, biosciences, sociology, and science and technology studies.

Sarah Franklin FBA, FAcSS, FRSB holds the Chair of Sociology at the University of Cambridge where she is also a Fellow of Christ's College. She is the founding Director of the Reproductive Sociology Research Group (ReproSoc) and co-Chair of Cambridge Reproduction. She is the author of *Embodied Progress: a cultural account of assisted conception* (1997, 2022) as well as numerous other publications on the social and cultural implications of new reproductive and genetic technologies.

Emily Jackson is a Professor of Law at the London School of Economics and Political Science, where she teaches Medical Law. She was a Member of the Human Fertilisation and Embryology Authority from 2003–2012, and its Deputy Chair from 2008–2012. She is a Fellow of the British Academy and was a Judicial Appointments Commissioner from 2014–2017.

The 14 Day Rule and Human Embryo Research

A Sociology of Biological Translation

Sarah Franklin and Emily Jackson

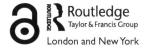

Routledge
Taylor & Francis Group
London and New York

Designed cover image: Human embryo, artwork – stock illustration,
© Getty Images. JUAN GARTNER

First published 2024
by Routledge
4 Park Square, Milton Park, Abingdon, Oxon OX14 4RN

and by Routledge
605 Third Avenue, New York, NY 10158

Routledge is an imprint of the Taylor & Francis Group, an informa business

British Library Cataloguing-in-Publication Data
A catalogue record for this book is available from the British Library

Library of Congress Cataloging-in-Publication Data
Names: Franklin, Sarah, 1960– author. | Jackson, Emily, 1966– author.
Title: The 14 day rule and human embryo research : a sociology of
biological translation / Sarah Franklin and Emily Jackson.
Other titles: Fourteen day rule and human embryo research
Description: Abingdon, Oxon ; New York, NY : Routledge, 2024. |
Includes bibliographical references and index.
Identifiers: LCCN 2024004396 (print) | LCCN 2024004397 (ebook) |
ISBN 9781032277905 (hardback) | ISBN 9781032277899 (paperback) |
ISBN 9781003294108 (ebook)
Subjects: LCSH: Human embryo—Research—Government policy—
Great Britain. | Human embryo—Research—Moral and ethical aspects. |
Embryology, Human—Research—Moral and ethical aspects.
Classification: LCC QM608 .F73 2024 (print) | LCC QM608 (ebook) |
DDC 612.6/4—dc23/eng/20240403
LC record available at https://lccn.loc.gov/2024004396
LC ebook record available at https://lccn.loc.gov/2024004397

ISBN: 978-1-032-27790-5 (hbk)
ISBN: 978-1-032-27789-9 (pbk)
ISBN: 978-1-003-29410-8 (ebk)

DOI: 10.4324/9781003294108

Typeset in Times New Roman
by codeMantra

To Anne and Mary, for their pioneering work and the example they set to us all.

Contents

Figures

Foreword

This book is a timely and detailed consideration of one of the most important legal issues in assisted human reproductive technology; namely the prohibition by law of keeping a human embryo *in vitro* for longer than 14 days and limiting its use in research to that time period.

First promoted by the influential UK Commission of Enquiry into Human Fertilisation and Embryology in 1984 under the chairmanship of Mary Warnock, this 'rule' was incorporated into legislation in the UK by the 1990 Human Fertilisation and Embryology Act. Despite the 'rule' being enforced by primary legislation in only a handful of other countries, it seems to have been accepted in practice for scientific research not to proceed past this objectively identifiable point. Although some restriction may have been due to national funding agencies not being prepared to fund work beyond this point, it is remarkable that with the huge proliferation of IVF in the private treatment market and venture capital sector that, as far as we are aware, this limit has been strictly adhered to voluntarily and globally for over 30 years.

The remarkable advances in IVF technology and our increasing understanding of early human embryology; the appearance of an array of powerful genomic techniques that allow the DNA of gametes and early embryos to be altered in ways that are heritable for multiple generations – germline genome editing; and the recent demonstration that various embryo-like constructs (embryoids, blastoids and gastruloids) can be made from stem cells *in vitro* that mimic human embryos during their early stages of development (so-called embryo models), have meant that the 14 day limit is now being challenged as never before. Whilst it is not the stated aim of researchers in this field that any of these new techniques would be used for construction of embryos destined for reproductive purposes, the same cannot be said for the use of *in vitro* derived gametes, which may have a role to play in alleviating intractable infertility. Before any of these techniques are considered for clinical use it is essential that the basic science is understood and safety evaluated, which will require the study of the 'embryo' beyond 14 days. Indeed it is during these later stages that many of the most profound changes in early development occur, and which, if they go awry, can lead to miscarriage or structural or genetic abnormality – thus making of them important clinical issues that are crying out for good research that is currently prohibited by the 14 day rule.

The 14 day rule and the use of human stem cells are consequently undergoing a thorough re-evaluation by the International Society for Stem Cell Research (ISSCR) which has called for a partial suspension of the limit based on the advantages of an extended time for such research. Similarly, the UK regulator, the Human Fertilisation and Embryology Authority, completed a consultation exercise in 2023 on modifying the current Act that includes a further consideration of the 14 day limit.

The two authors of this volume, who I admire immensely and have worked with personally for many years, are highly experienced, complementary experts in the law and social consequences of assisted reproduction. In this book they deal confidently and expertly with this fraught area. I was particularly pleased to see that in chapter 3, they give appropriate recognition to the remarkable Dr Anne McLaren who was the rational scientific voice on the Warnock Commission that eventually led to 14 days being accepted as a reasoned and reasonable limit. The book is a highly readable and unique work that is perfectly timed to coincide with the pressure for change and for the legal and social machinations that will follow.

Peter Braude OBE MA PhD FMedSci FRCOG FRSB
Emeritus Professor in Obstetrics and Gynaecology, King's College
London and Former Director of the Assisted Conception Unit,
and Centre for Preimplantation Genetic Diagnosis,
Guy's and St Thomas' NHS Hospital Foundation Trust

Acknowledgements

This book has a longer history than might appear to be the case given that extending the 14 day rule has only recently become a subject of serious international discussion. Funding for the research that informs this book was provided by the Welcome Trust, the British Academy, the University of Cambridge, the Economic and Social Research Council (UKRI) and the LSE. Many of our colleagues have been hugely helpful in refining our arguments including Robin Lovell-Badge, Peter Rugg Gunn, Kathy Niakan and Kathy Liddell. We are especially grateful to Sandy Starr, Sarah Norcross and Peter Braude for detailed readings of the penultimate draft. All responsibility for the final arguments is of course ours alone. We also want to thank Rob Doubleday of the Centre for Science Policy and Christina Roziek from Cambridge Reproduction for organising the hugely helpful discussion meetings about the governance of stem-cell based embryo models at Cambridge in the summer and autumn of 2023. Finally, we are very grateful to Anne McLaren's family – Susan, Jonathan and Caroline – for helping us with illustrations. In 2016, the staff of the Department of Health Repository in Burnley was essential in locating the original Warnock files (after a ten year search), and these have proven vital to understanding the evolution of the original 14 day rule proposals. Cambridge University Press generously enables reprinting of material published in their journal, including much of the material in Chapter 3 that was originally published as 'Developmental Landmarks' in 2019 in the CUP journal *Contemporary Studies in Society and History*. We are especially grateful to the Routledge/Taylor and Francis editorial and production team, in particular our hugely helpful editor Grace McInnes, as well as Amy Thomson, Isabel Voice, Louise Ingham, Hamish Ironside, Bonita Glanville-Morris and Miriam Pilcher-Clayton.

1 What is the 14 Day Rule and Why Does it Matter?

In this book we address a very specific subject, yet one that encapsulates many of the most important questions concerning the future of biomedicine, its governance and the social contract that connects them – because these are what the story of the 14 day rule is all about. The following chapters explore why this unique piece of legislation matters to us all, and so we start with some very basic questions. What is the 14 day rule and why is it important? What are its origins and histories, and why does its future matter to the general public, as well as to governments around the world? Why are scientists and policy makers so concerned about this question? And above all why should it matter to you? In this book we offer several different answers to these questions that bring us into conversation with many different players, disciplines, organisations and proposals. Our journey takes us back in time to how the 14 day rule was originally established and looks forward to consider what its future might – or might not – be. But first let's answer two of the most important questions: what is the 14 day rule and why are we writing this book?

The simplest way to describe the 14 day rule is that it is a pivotal policy within a wider regulatory structure governing 'human fertilisation and embryology' in the UK, set up by the Human Fertilisation and Embryology (HFE) Act 1990, and administered by the Human Fertilisation and Embryology Authority (HFEA).[1] The 14 day rule establishes the maximum period of time for which embryos can be cultured *in vitro*.[2] If embryos are frozen for future use, the clock 'stops' because the embryos are effectively frozen in time, and will not develop further until they are thawed.

We will revisit the story of how the HFE Act came into being in later sections of this book, and this will tell us much more about why the 14 day rule was so important to that legislation, but for now it is enough to explain simply that the 14 day rule functions as a prohibition – a red line that can't be crossed in human embryo research. This line might appear to be a relatively simple regulatory mechanism – and indeed that is in some ways both the secret of its success and part of its ongoing regulatory appeal. However, as we shall see, the question of 'where to draw the line' between permissible and impermissible research was one of the most challenging and complex hurdles that needed to be faced by Britain's famous Warnock Committee, who placed this important literal, symbolic and definitive line at the centre of their legislative proposals.

DOI: 10.4324/9781003294108-1

Perhaps uniquely in regulatory policy governing bioscience, the UK's 14 day rule governing human embryo research, which was initially drafted 40 years ago, is at once the essence of simplicity and a highly complex piece of legislation. It is a bright clear line and an amalgam, or even, as we shall see, an enigma. Unsurprisingly, the members of the Warnock Committee tasked with delivering a coherent system of regulation for the legal *terra nullius* of human embryology sought to establish a firm basis on which to enact new laws that would set clear parameters around the unprecedented clinical and research possibilities opened up by successful human IVF. They needed, however, two rather different ingredients to meet the high bar of public, professional and parliamentary scrutiny. The upper time limit for permissible research on human embryos which served as a cornerstone for a strict national licensing system needed to be based on absolute scientific certainty about the precise stages of embryological development, and thus had to be firmly grounded in well-characterised and undisputed biological 'landmarks'. On the other hand, to be enforceable, pragmatic and sustainable as a regulatory mechanism, the law had to be readily applied and easily enforced by regulators, in every IVF clinic and affiliated research lab across the entire country. The law therefore also had to offer a simplified means of translating precise embryological facts into clear bright lines.

Initially, the Committee sought to identify a key point in embryological development where a natural, biological dividing line could be identified, and, as we shall see in Chapter 3, they pointed to the formation of the embryonic disc, or primitive streak, at approximately day 14 of early human development. This is indeed a key stage in development, when several definitive transformations converge in the emergence of a new individual. These changes can be interpreted to distinguish two key embryological entities – the blastocyst and the gastrula. As the developing blastocyst begins to attach to the uterine lining, a flat disc forms that will become the axis of a single body plan. This axis is the first formative alignment that marks the onset of gastrulation – the transformation of a flat, two-dimensional embryonic disc into the three-dimensional tube that will eventually become the inside of the developing body (*gastrula* comes from the Greek word for 'stomach'). The axial dividing line of this new individual body plan is considered a developmental landmark, known as the 'primitive streak', and indeed appears as a faint groove, or trough, as the two sides of the developing gastrula curl inwards.

Definitive as this landmark embryological event might be, however, it was not enough by itself to provide the basis for legislation. Development is a continuous process: it is not neatly punctuated by singular events. Moreover, regulators could not be expected to inspect every embryo under a microscope and not all gastrulation events are identically timed. A primitive streak might not form until day 15, for example, and who would be keeping track? Thus although it initially appeared logical to base the law on a natural, biological 'fact' of embryological development, this proved too elusive. To enable regulation, a simple translation was devised by setting a 14 day limit. As Mary Warnock noted with characteristic pragmatism, 14 days is a limit everyone can easily recognise – no specialist training or equipment is needed to count 14 days on a calendar. At the same time, the limit remains at least partially based on observable and established biological fact, and thus can't be accused of being entirely arbitrary. This translation of a clear biological 'line' into a numeric 14 day limit had other advantages too. As we shall see, it enabled the post 14 day developing embryo to be designated as a new and separate entity – namely 'the embryo proper', referring to the part of the embryo that would become a new individual as opposed to the supporting tissues and nutrients, including the placenta. The embryo prior to this point could thus also acquire a new status, as the 'pre-embryo' – referring to the period before 14 days.

Altogether, this new embryological roadmap gave the Warnock Committee exactly what it needed to establish a robust, enforceable, persuasive and non-arbitrary limit for human embryo research. Above all, this firm limit clearly communicated a crucial principle: human embryo research could be permitted, but only on a strictly limited and highly regulated basis. Moreover, the 14 day rule not only established a clear bright line between permissible and impermissible research but offered a viable, attractive and credible means of enforcing it. For the purpose of presenting their regulatory proposals to Parliament, the professional scientific community, journalists and the general public, the 14 day rule established the basis for accommodating the widest range of views: research would be allowed but also controlled, the law would be objectively grounded in textbook embryology but not indecipherably or impractically so. The limit combined a biological line, a legal line and a regulatory line but also a simple timeline, and thus a clear and credible enforcement mechanism. In the end, the 14 day rule and its persuasive amalgamation of principled but pragmatic, strict but permissive, and cautious but progressive elements proved not only key to the success of the Human Fertilisation and Embryology Bill that resulted from the Warnock Committee's efforts, but also became the 1990 HFE Act's signature component, symbolic anchor and most widely emulated feature worldwide. So successful was the recombinant logic of the 14 day rule that in the three decades since its passage into statute it has not only become the most famous and widely replicated feature of the UK's HFE Act, but the *de facto* global regulatory standard for human embryo research, with nearly identical laws having been passed by 12 other countries (Matthews and Moralí 2020), and its even wider application as 'soft law' or guidance.

One of the main reasons so many countries have copied the UK's example in implementing 14 day rules of their own is because no other legislature has ever managed to regulate 'human fertilisation and embryology' as comprehensively as the UK Parliament. The story of how the UK Parliament managed this singular feat is more complex than this book can accommodate, but is partly told in Chapters 4 and 5.[3] However, it should immediately become apparent that two of the main reasons why the 14 day rule is so consequential are that it is now the default global regulatory policy for controversial bioscience involving human embryo-based methodologies, and that legislation in this area is notoriously difficult to enact.

The 14 day rule is famous for another reason too, however, which, as already noted above, is the central role it played in the design of the what became the HFE Act, and in the lengthy deliberations of the committee that proposed it, chaired by the eminent philosopher Mary Warnock. When the Warnock Report was published in 1984, it contained 64 recommendations resulting from a two year consultation process that eventually formed the basis for the HFE Bill, enacted in 1990. When we look in more detail at how the proposals which became legislation were originally formulated by the Warnock Committee (Chapter 3), we will note yet another key feature of the 14 day rule, notably that in addition to being an amalgam of different systems of reasoning it was also a compromise based on a sociological principle of exchange, or reciprocity: *in exchange* for allowing valuable research into human embryology and reproduction, including new techniques such as IVF, any such research would be subject to the very highest level of scrutiny, require a licence and be overseen by a specialist independent public authority. Likewise, *in return* for allowing such research to proceed, the public could benefit from steady progress in the improvement not only of IVF and other assisted conception technologies, but basic research into human embryology and development.

Crucially, it is this element of compromise articulated through a language of exchange that explains why the 14 day rule has gained such a prominent status in the fast-paced and highly controversial arenas of reproductive research, technology and regulation of translational bioscience, where this rule stands virtually alone as an example of not only strict-but-permissive but also enduring and resilient legislation. We explore this unique legacy further in Chapter 5, where we look in more detail at Warnock's decision to place a compromise solution at the heart of her legislative strategy, and why this has proven to be so remarkably successful. After all, not only was this strategy largely responsible for the success of the Warnock Committee in devising a viable legislative blueprint in 1984 (all 64 of the Committee's original recommendations were eventually enacted into law in 1990), but the enduring legacy of this robust-but-permissive legislation has in turn enabled what has been described as the 'Warnock Consensus' (Jasanoff and Metzler 2020), referring to both the stability of the Warnock formula as a statutory anchor for subsequent amendments to the Human Fertilisation and Embryology Act and the unusually favourable environment for innovative biomedical research it has supported in the UK for more than three decades.

This favourable climate for biomedical research has in turn been enabled not only by the UK's uniquely cautious-but-progressive legislative infrastructure for the governance of human fertilisation and embryology but by an unusually high degree of public support. In a recent comment on the Warnock Consensus, American and German political scientists Sheila Jasanoff and Ingrid Metzler, who coined this term, observe with admiration that a whole host of controversial biomedical innovations including human embryonic stem cell research, preimplantation genetic testing (PGT, or in tabloid terms, 'designer babies'), somatic cell nuclear transfer ('cloning'), mitochondrial donation ('three parent babies') and even 'human admixed embryos' – in which various combinations of human and animal material can be used both clinically[4] and for research purposes– have all proceeded 'markedly more smoothly [in the UK] than in other Western nations' (Jasanoff and Metzler 2020: 16). Moreover, they observe, the unusual degree of public consensus over the permissibility of such controversial procedures in the UK appears to have occurred *because of* the extensive public consultation to which they were subjected, rather than in spite of it. In marked contrast to 'the political uproar or political deadlock that characterized comparable debates in Germany and the United States' (and many other countries), greater public engagement with controversial issues such as genetic testing of embryos, third party DNA donation for reproductive purposes and even the use of animal eggs as 'incubators' to grow new human cells and the creation of human admixed embryos for research (Royal Society 2008) appears to have facilitated successful pursuit *and* comprehensive regulation of these areas in the UK – rather than impeding them.

'Virtuous circles' of this kind are rare in both legislative and policy terms, but even more so in emotive areas such as scientific research and clinical applications affecting the very earliest stages of human development, the manipulation of human embryos *in vitro*, and assisted conception. It has been noted by many observers in the UK Parliament, as well as policy makers worldwide, that the enduring regulatory infrastructure enabled by Warnock's astute foresight, guidance and strategic chairing of her Committee is a 'unicorn' achievement in ethical, social and political as well as legislative terms. As is now even more evident in retrospect, 40 years after the publication of her Committee's original Report, Warnock's ultimate and lasting achievement has been to establish public confidence in an area many seasoned observers understandably perceived as too divisive for any consensual governance structure ever to be established at all, never mind one that could be successfully maintained, updated and repeatedly amended over several decades. Most remarkable of all is the strong link between widespread public understanding of, respect for and consequent willingness to support even quite radically innovative techniques such as human admixed embryos. As Dame Suzi Leather, a former Chair of the Human Fertilisation and Embryology Authority, commented in 2018: '[P]erhaps the greatest achievement of the Warnock committee is that it managed to get an ethical consensus that people understood as well as shared' (HL Deb 13 September 2018).

The crucial issue of public trust brings us to the three final reasons the 14 day rule offers a unique case study in policy, governance and regulation related to human reproduction and embryology, for this is indeed an issue that Mary Warnock and her equally astute and influential scientific advisor, Dr Anne McLaren, understood with remarkable depth and prescience. It is here, in relation to the importance of public trust to translational science more widely, that we argue the lessons of the 14 day rule are especially relevant today, amidst ever more complex public debate over issues such as the use of human gene editing for reproductive purposes, the creation of stem-cell derived gametes and the emergence of highly advanced human embryo models that closely mimic the very earliest stages of human development. These debates remind us that the deep respect for public trust in science shared between Warnock and McLaren was not only pivotal to their success as communicators and policy architects, but was rooted in a highly unusual combination of intuitive, pragmatic and sociological insights. These were in turn the same insights that informed the key principles that guided both the deliberation process and the final recommendations of the Warnock Committee. As Warnock herself stated in her original Report:

> People generally want some principles or other to govern the development and use of the new techniques. There must be some barriers that are not crossed, some limits fixed beyond which people must not be allowed to go. A society which had no inhibiting limits, especially in the areas of birth and death, of the setting up of families and the valuing of human life, would be a society without moral scruples, *and this nobody wants.*
>
> (Warnock 1984: para. 5.5, emphasis added)

This simple principle, that *some legislation is preferable to none* in areas of great moral importance to society, is typical of the kind of axiom Warnock placed at the heart of her project to design legislation that would be pragmatic, popular and workable, as well as clearly articulated, logically coherent and grounded on firm moral reasoning. This 'Warnockian' approach to legislation skilfully balances the essential requirement for an enforceable line to be definitely drawn against the necessity for compromise about where, exactly, it will be. It becomes a logical consequence that some flexibility around what the limits should be, exactly, will be required in order to achieve the greater good of having any limits at all. Crucially, however, the moral weight of this principle lies in achieving the responsible and laudable social goal, on behalf of everyone, of establishing 'some barriers that are not crossed' rather than determining which barriers or limits these are, exactly.

To some, this is quite simply an 'ends justifies the means', or familiar utilitarian argument.[5] But Warnock's pragmatism was not merely instrumental: it originated in a sense, and definition, of moral purpose – and in particular sought to express social morality through the law – by establishing lines that can't be crossed. Such rules, to Warnock – a Head Teacher for much of her career as well as a philosopher by training – were not simply lines of prohibition: respect for agreed and established limits embodied something larger and more positive, namely the value of confirming reciprocal social obligations and duties, expressed as mutual responsibilities to each other, and articulated as both the individual and institutional values that bind us together. For Warnock, then, the 'end' of creating a protective barrier around the sensitive and emotive topic of human embryo research was a pragmatic policy goal, but nonetheless *primarily the expression of a moral principle* to which the idea of society as a collective moral force was paramount. To Warnock, laws were not only literal but also expressive, emblematic and representative – she argued that having a law rather than no law on a matter of great moral consequence 'stands for the moral idea of society itself' (Warnock 1985).

The critique of this position has long been that it can justify somewhat arbitrary laws, and this was a criticism Warnock both accepted and rejected, arguing in response that laws are indeed often arbitrary – for example, driving on the left- or right-hand side of the road – and hence can be changed. She argued, logically, that arbitrariness is not an absolute position, and that not all laws that are partially arbitrary are entirely so. In this respect as well as in her understanding of morality,

Warnock's reasoning takes on a distinctively sociological character, in that her priority was to use the law to achieve a social and moral good by avoiding a legal vacuum. Hers was in many ways a very precise and backwards-focussed logic that begins where her quotation above ends, namely with *what 'nobody wants'*. This is a crucially important feature of Warnock's reasoning, as we shall see, because, somewhat paradoxically, the entire edifice of legislation built around the strategic compromise of a somewhat arbitrary 14 day limit on embryo research is designed with a negative outcome in mind – of avoiding ending up without any legislation at all.

Tellingly, this is by far the most common scenario worldwide. Of the nearly 200 countries on the planet, only a handful have any legislation at all related to human embryo research, and none other than Britain has anything like comprehensive legislation in this area.

This brings us to the question of why we are writing this book? Yes, we are a sociology and a law professor, and we have both written extensively about the Warnock Report and reproductive regulation. We worked together at the LSE for many years and have remained close colleagues ever since. Emily has direct experience of the HFEA as its former deputy chair and the added experience of many cognate committee memberships. Sarah has conducted extensive qualitative research on many of the techniques covered by the HFEA, including IVF, PGT, human embryo research, cloning and stem cell technology. We have both published extensively about the 14 day rule, and like many people who work in the broad interdisciplinary field of research on new reproductive technologies we are consequently very aware of how much is at stake in potentially changing it. To both of us, and as we stated at the outset of this chapter, the 14 day rule offers a vital and unique object lesson for a much wider set of questions about how biogovernance should be understood as we move ever more deeply into questions about what limits that are needed to safeguard and enable successful biological translation. The question of changing the 14 day rule, in other words, recapitulates the age old question of how to *beneficially limit* scientific and technological research?

And so we return to the key question of whether the 14 day rule need to be changed, and, if so, why? Clearly there are significant risks to abandoning a law that is not only highly successful but has become an enduring symbol of society's ability to set firm limits on controversial scientific research. Over 40 years, however, the reasons why such a successful example of regulatory policy might need to be revisited have accumulated. To begin with, and perhaps most obviously, culturing embryos beyond 14 days has only recently become a viable scientific possibility, and so in some ways the question of whether or not it should be permissible was irrelevant until 2016 when the first techniques for more extended human embryo culture were developed by scientists in Cambridge, London and New York (Deglincerti et al. 2016; Shahbazi et al. 2016). In the wake of these discoveries a number of new scientific possibilities emerged, and they have been joined by others leading to widespread calls for new legislation (Foreman et al. 2023; Hengstschläger and Rosner 2021). In addition to the ability to culture embryos *in vitro* for longer, the successful derivation of functional human gametes from stem cells, and the creation of advanced embryo-like models and brain organoids, led the International

Society for Stem Cell Research (ISSCR) to develop new guidelines for stem cell research and clinical translation in 2021. They also recommended that there should be 'public conversations', not only about the 'scientific significance' of research on embryos beyond 14 days, but also its 'societal and ethical issues'. Already we have seen the first public engagement exercises begin to take place on these issues here in the UK, and we discuss the early findings from these exercises, and what they might suggest about the future of legislation in this area, in Chapter 7.

The future of the 14 day rule has become a particularly important question due to the huge range of embryoid, embryo-like, embryo-derived and embryogenic entities that are now involved in an increasingly wide range of scientific research programmes worldwide. We discuss these further at the end of this book, but for now the important point is that these new means of modelling, replicating, imitating and thus better understanding the basic generative and regenerative processes of biological development – especially in humans – has huge translational importance. By 'translational' we refer to the process of 'translating' basic scientific research into successful applications, such as new health benefits and better diagnoses and treatment for disease. Coupled with newfound abilities to derive, differentiate, direct, reprogramme, and redesign cell lines and organoids that recapitulate existing morphology (and pathology), a major paradigm shift is taking place in both bioscience and biomedicine. Newly acquired experimental methods for successfully growing complex living entities and systems *in vitro* that model actual living tissues and their functions – such as pancreatic, kidney or skin cell lines and organoids – offer new pathways for not only treating but ultimately curing widespread chronic disease such as diabetes. In their original form, all of these cells and organs have a single source, namely the human embryo, and as a result the ability to harness this unique source of totipotent cellular vitality has gained increasing importance to the contemporary life sciences.

Human embryonic stem cells were not successfully derived until the close of the twentieth century and initial treatment protocols have had limited success to date (Golchin et al. 2021). However, both stem cell science and tissue engineering, alongside regenerative medicine, are new fields and their 'translational pipeline' holds many promising leads. These will not only open the door to new clinical therapies, but will help to confirm, standardise and more finely tune existing cellular regeneration technologies – including new methods of creating reproductive and embryonic cells *in vitro* (as was announced in June of 2023). All of these developments will not only have translational significance for health care and for bioscience. They will also change what people understand an embryo to be, especially as the lines are now blurring between so-called synthetic, artificial and 'unassisted' embryos – just as the lines have already blurred between IVF and 'unassisted' conception, or between cells and stem cells, or cell lines and organoids (Ball 2023).

These changes to public perceptions of embryos in relation to new experimental methods in translational biology have now been developing for several decades. In the 1990s the cloning of Dolly the sheep led to the widespread circulation of images of microinjection of cells (somatic cell nuclear transfer) and a worldwide debate about the possibility of human cloning. In the early noughties, the derivation of human embryonic stem cell lines and therapeutic cloning similarly led to widespread media coverage of *in vitro* human embryo micromanipulation using tiny glass pipettes. These projects were linked to the emergence of the new field of regenerative medicine, through which absent or malfunctioning cells and tissues linked to diseases such as diabetes, cardiac arrythmia or diabetes could be grown *in vitro* and transplanted into affected patients. In a pathbreaking project led by Professor Doug Melton at Harvard's Stem Cell Institute aimed at curing childhood diabetes, scientists returned to square one by harnessing *in vitro* embryonic cell lines to develop functional pancreatic Beta cells. Once these were successfully derived, and functional, the scientists turned to clinicians to begin trialling the introduction of these cells into affected patients. Working with Boston's famous Joslin Diabetes Center, they are now trialling ways to transplant these cells into patients with the goal of creating as cure for diabetes – a disease that affects 10% of the American population.

New insights derived from embryo research such as those mentioned above are thus part of a long series of changes in the transformation of the human embryo into a vital research 'window' – and also tool – for translational and regenerative research (Franklin 2013a, 2013b, 2013c). These new *in vitro* techniques involving embryonic cells, cell lines and models are now rapidly accelerating scientists' abilities to understand fundamental developmental processes, as well as key stages in embryonic development such as implantation. Cultured embryonic systems, entities and models derived from donated human embryos have now been complemented by *in vitro* models wholly derived from experimentally cultured stem cells, which closely replicate normal development and thus offer the possibility to observe previously inaccessible aspects of the crucial sequence of formative events at the earliest stages of human life. In labs such as those of Jacob Hanna in Israel, Nicolas Rivron in Austria and Magdalena Zernicka-Goetz, Kathy Niakan and Naomi Moris in the UK, teams are now proposing to use insights from embryo modelling to explore why and how some pregnancies fail, and to identify the causes of birth defects and diseases – explorations which could yield better diagnoses as well as treatments, but also better understandings of how the embryo develops within the womb.

Now that it is not only possible to culture human embryos for more than 14 days but is also increasingly clear how many scientific and clinical benefits could be achieved by extending the 14 day limit, there is inevitably a more pressing question as to whether such an extension is justified, and what kind of line could be drawn in its place. In Chapter 6 we review these arguments in depth, and in Chapter 7 we provide an overview of several possible routes forward. In the wake of the worldwide headlines accompanying the announcement of the creation of new embryo models in 2023, the question of how best to update the regulation of 'human fertilisation and embryology' took on even greater significance, leading to more urgent calls for social, ethical and legislative debate as well as more robust public consultation. Increasingly the concern expressed by many leading scientific researchers in this field is that as science begins to outpace existing legislation, a new legal vacuum is emerging – with potential hazards for social trust in science, as well as for science itself.

Much as new legislation may be needed, however, abandoning the 14 day rule, which has stood the test of time as not only as a guiding principle of regulation but as a mechanism for promoting public trust in the governance of controversial bioscientific innovation, is not without its dangers. For many years before her death in 2019, Mary Warnock consistently expressed significant reservations about lifting the anchor that has secured the UK's widely respected HFEA through so many storms so far. But she did not rule out this possibility completely. She urged extreme caution as the downsides of overturning well-established regulatory principles and guidelines are fairly obvious. Reopening a debate that was considered by many to be irreconcilable is one obvious hazard. The singularity of the British achievement in creating a highly regulated research environment for translational biomedicine that is also highly permissive and stable is another, and the degree of public trust in this system is perhaps the most vulnerable of all to any sudden shifts or new directions.

The main reason, then, why we are writing this book is because we are now in the midst of a new discussion about the future of human embryo research, which is very different from the one that began in 1978 with the birth of Louise Brown. In the 1970s, the idea that conception could take place in a Petri dish in a lab, and produce a 'test tube baby' was profoundly new and shocking. Although IVF itself is now commonplace and routine, more recent scientific developments – such as the creation of embryo models – or 'stembryos' – and brain organoids – are less so, and may require new lines to be drawn in order to reassure the public, and to ensure a stable environment for scientific research. When trying to work out what can legitimately be done with these new entities, the Warnock approach to the regulation of cutting-edge research continues to stand as a salutary lesson in communication, compromise and translation. The importance of two-way public engagement, and the drawing of clear and bright regulatory lines in order to engender public confidence is as important today as it was four decades ago.

As scholars who have worked in this field for many decades, we hope this book can be helpful in laying out some of the many important frameworks that have been developed for the analysis of reproductive research, technology and innovation. Like Mary Warnock, we also argue that there are a number of approaches that are not very helpful, and may even best be avoided, in the effort to determine how best to establish governance around 'human fertilisation and embryology' in the future. Approaches, for example, which begin by attempting to definitively establish the absolute moral and ethical qualities of human embryos are very challenging to work with, both because they are so difficult (if not impossible) to specify and because they generate such visceral disagreement. Similarly, arguments about what embryos essentially 'are' – ontologically or biologically – lead to endless disagreements about which are the main, or most important properties or criteria that need to be take into account. As we have already seen, the seemingly obvious tactic of trying to identify distinct natural, biological, developmental or morphological characteristics in order to determine where lines should be drawn is much more difficult than it appears, and it is even more difficult to establish limits on the basis of embryonic potential. The same problem occurs when definitions of what is 'special' about the human embryo evoke extended temporal frames, such as the argument that every conceptus is a potential human being.

Our preference in this book, and one of the guiding principles we offer, is that we need increasingly to be aware of the extremely broad range of living human entities that now fall into the categories of embryoid, embryo-like, embryogenic and embryonic. This means it makes sense to focus on permissible and impermissible uses of embryos, agreed or prohibited research objectives and codes of conduct for new fields of enquiry rather than the intrinsic qualities of novel biological entities such as 'stembryos'. Likewise, we need to be careful to specify not only the sources of such entities, and how they are created or made, but also what purposes they are intended to serve, for whom, and under what specific conditions. We need robust social processes for biogovernance that can reliably lead to transparent, enforceable and consensual guidelines – and these need to involve high levels of public consultation as well as effective two-way communication between the scientific community and the general public. Establishing beneficial limits for controversial scientific research also requires effective cooperation between government, science and industry – as well as policy makers, legislators and public engagement specialists. A final point we need to pay increasing attention to is the importance of science communication, including how terms like 'artificial', 'synthetic' and even 'embryonic' are used. Embryo models, for example, are increasingly well characterised in terms of their lineage, provenance, appearance, metabolism and behaviour – but they also differ hugely in kind, type and uses. Very large-scale populations of dish-derived embryo-like entities created for experimental purposes differ significantly, for example, from frozen fertilised eggs in an IVF lab. Since we are in many ways at the very beginning of developing a new social contract for reproductive bioscience, we do not offer specific answers to the question of, for example, what any future time limit on embryo research might be. Moreover, as we suggest in our conclusion, this might not even be the main question we need to be asking – and it is certainly not the only one. But what we do offer is a review of important lessons that have already been learned from the 14 day rule and its legacies.

Inevitably, since it is being written in the midst of so much change and uncertainty, this book is less concerned with precisely answering the question of what legislative mechanisms might be needed in the future than establishing a framework for approaching that question, in terms of what we might need to know, who we might need to ask, and where we might look for examples to guide us. One of our main arguments is that such a framework must take into account the broad sociological changes that affect translational science as well as the specific challenges of highly technical new fields such as embryo modelling. As well as taking into account issues such as the diversification of the meaning of 'embryo research', or even 'human embryo', that we have seen over the past 40 years since the first human egg was successfully fertilised *in vitro* in 1968, we also need to take into account the enormous changes affecting perceptions of biology, technology and society that have resulted from the rapid spread of IVF-based technologies over the past half century. These technologies, including stem cell research, cloning, gametogenesis and embryo modelling have emerged side-by-side with a huge and burgeoning fertility industry that has ushered in a number of very important shifts in public perceptions of both biology and bioscience that should not be underestimated. These include the social facts that most people now understand IVF as an acceptable and routine way to have a baby, and that research on both human and animal embryos plays a well-established and vital role in experimental scientific progress in a wide range of sectors – from agriculture and the study of human aging to fertility care and regenerative medicine. Put even more bluntly, both the translational success of IVF and the promises of human-embryo derived stem cell therapy have changed how people understand 'the facts of life' – namely that the very earliest stages of embryonic development hold the keys to human biological repair. And, furthermore, that these repairs can be nothing short of revolutionary – as the now approximately 10 million 'miracle babies' born from IVF worldwide have confirmed over the past half century.

As we approach the second quarter of the twenty-first century, it is the very fact that IVF has become so unremarkable that most definitively confirms how much it has transformed perceptions of technologically assisted biology. It is for the same reason no exaggeration to claim that IVF is one of the most successful translational technologies of the twentieth century and that it has substantially transformed the way in which human reproduction is both practiced and imagined. But it is equally true that this transformation is as yet quite poorly documented or understood in large part due to the longstanding neglect of issues related to human reproduction in traditional accounts of modern industrial society and the impact of science and technology.

A key argument of this book is that taking a broad sociological look at the effects on public perceptions of bioscience of the normalisation of human fertility technology, and in particular IVF, over the past half century is both overdue and essential. There is a huge difference, for example, between public perceptions of *in vitro* human embryos today and in 1982 when Mary Warnock sat down to discuss them with her committee. It is worth remembering too, especially as it might easily be forgotten in today's IVF-ified society, that for many observers the most likely outcome of the formal establishment of a Committee of Inquiry into human fertilisation and embryology in the wake of the world's first birth of a baby following IVF and embryo transfer (ET) in 1978 would have been the banning of both techniques. Indeed, such a ban was very nearly put in place in 1985, following a majority vote in the UK Parliament of 238 to 66 opponents (a ratio of more than 3 to 1) in favour of Enoch Powell's Unborn Children (Protection) Bill, which would have criminalised all human embryo research and thus effectively have brought an end to IVF treatment as well. It would also have had the unprecedented effect of rendering illegal two ongoing Medical Research Council (MRC)-funded research projects.

As the sociologist Michael Mulkay (1997) points out in his comprehensive study of the embryo research debate that took place in the UK in the 1980s, Enoch Powell was not an anti-abortion politician and had never been active in issues relation to issues of this kind previously. His Bill was not ideologically motivated but populist. He was convinced to introduce his Bill, he said, because he had discovered that his own 'deep feeling of moral repugnance' about embryo research was widely shared 'among all classes and callings and throughout the people of this country' (quoted in Mulkay 1997: 28). As many other commentators have noted[6], it was in no small part the shock of the very sizeable majority of parliamentary opposition to human embryo research, accompanied by subsequent opinion polls showing that fewer than a third of adult British citizens supported such research (ibid.: 29), that galvanised a major campaign to change public opinion. Crucial to this campaign was the argument that without embryo research there could be no IVF treatment for infertility nor preimplantation testing for serious genetic disease.

The imminent threat the Powell Bill posed to MRC-funded research on embryos led the MRC to support the creation of an action group – the Professional Advisory Group for Infertility and Genetic Services (PAGIGS) – to work with sympathetic MPs in order to ensure 'that there were members of the group available, day and night, to provide advice and scribble briefs for MPs' (Braude 2009). Chaired by Peter Braude, PAGIGS' membership included Anne McLaren, Martin Johnson and Robert Winston, and it ensured that the scientific community in the UK learned the lesson that scientists have an essential role to play in shaping regulation. As Braude (2009) has put it, 'to be effective in this role they must accept that speaking to the press and the public should be seen not as an egocentric indulgence to be avoided, but as part of the scientist's job'.

With the benefit of hindsight, the crucial lesson of the early reactions to the Warnock Report recommendations, including the 14 day limit on human embryo research, was that securing both parliamentary and public support would require, as repeated editorials in the prestigious scientific journal *Nature* urgently advised, making the case for the importance of such research to successful clinical applications. In turn, by succeeding in this effort, the UK established its influence as the home of the emergent IVF industry and, over the next three decades, as one of the world's most secure and well-regulated environments for translational biomedical research based on the IVF technique. Importantly, and perhaps with fitting Warnockian irony, it was the initial failure of the UK scientific community to accurately judge either public or parliamentary reaction to embryo research that catalysed the well-organised and energetic subsequent campaign to change hearts and minds. PAGIGS became the lead campaigning organisation PROGRESS, which brought together not only proponents of embryo research, but also patients, health professionals and infertility support groups. This organisation, renamed the Progress Educational Trust in 1992, continues four decades later to play a vital role in facilitating public dialogue and debate related to new forms of reproductive biomedicine (www.progress.org).

Understanding how IVF has transformed popular understandings of conception, fertility, biology and genetics (a.k.a. 'the facts of life') is important because these are also quite fundamental to common-sense ideas about many other things, from gender and technology to health, medicine and bioscience. One of the most important effects of IVF has not only been to destigmatise and normalise a more explicit, intimate and elaborate interaction between human reproduction and technology, but to embed the idea that *in vitro* fertilisation is essentially the same as natural *in vivo* conception as far as the ability to produce perfectly normal offspring is concerned. Although there are those who continue to object to IVF in principle, the increasingly taken-for-granted equivalence between assisted and unassisted reproduction has, over the past half century, helped to establish a new reproductive logic in which natural and technological reproduction increasingly overlap, and this new reproductive order is now an established fact of life (Franklin 2013a, 2022). This 'IVF effect' is one of several examples we offer in this book of sociological forces that are integral to translational bioscience, and one of the reasons why we argue that biological translation must be sociologically informed.

This brings us back to the basic connection that is so vitally important to understanding the social forces that shape translational bioscience, which is that technologies such as IVF are intimately interwoven with collective values that matter deeply to people, whether they are scientists or patients, parliamentarians or parents, members of the general public or medical professionals. These include values such as fairness, equity, trust, decency and civility. Such values are often closely linked to understandings of community, welfare and social belonging as well as of family obligations, parenting, kinship ties and thus also personal identity. As a future-orientated reproductive technology, IVF invokes a wide range of ethical questions and intergenerational obligations – including feelings of responsibility for future human societies, and the duty to alleviate human suffering, as well as the importance of having children and building families.

In sum, reproduction matters to people for reasons that inform but also supersede their personal reproductive choices. Self-evidently, few questions are as existential as whether or not to reproduce, or for that matter how, and this is one of the main reasons that technological assistance to reproduction has been seen by anthropologists such as Marilyn Strathern to introduce not only a new way of thinking about starting a family but a new perspective on the making of social connections more widely and indeed a new logic of life (Strathern 1992a, 1992b). Ideas about the naturalness of reproductive ties and their moral significance, while evoking strong opinions and feelings in themselves, are also used as idioms to represent other things – including culture, religion, tradition, nation and humanity. Indeed such references are ubiquitous, and this is one of the reasons it has long been an anthropological axiom that what people think and feel about reproduction tells you a great deal about what they think and feel about everything else.

The profoundly social question of what human reproduction means to people over and above simply having babies is one that Mary Warnock and her key scientific advisor, Anne McLaren, clearly placed at the heart of their ambitious project to devise a legislative and regulatory infrastructure that would both limit and support highly innovative biomedical research into human fertilisation and embryology. Much as the general public might not have even a remote awareness of gastrulation, they assumed that the proverbial passenger on the Clapham omnibus knew lots of other equally important facts about the human condition. As we shall see, part of their strategy was to assume people are already highly knowledgeable about both the role of science in society and its potential benefits in areas such as reproduction. They also made the somewhat unorthodox assumption that it not only matters that people know and understand the challenges of infertility, genetic disease, miscarriage and unwanted childlessness, but that it matters how they *feel* about them. The fact that these are subjects about which people have strong feelings was not only important to Warnock but a positive sign that the question of how society responds to them is morally important and socially binding.

As we shall see, all of these elements in the formation of the Warnock Consensus can helpfully be understood through a framework we are describing as a sociology of biological translation. Among the most important elements we discuss in relation to this concept is the crucial issue of public trust. Trust is emotional but also rational. It is relational and dialogic: trust is strengthened through being mutually reciprocated, and it is broken when expectations of reciprocity are disappointed, disrespected – or simply dispensed with altogether. In many ways what is most remarkable about the 14 day rule is the successful role it has played in *reinforcing public trust and confidence over time* by enabling controversial research to proceed within a clearly delimited, transparent, enforceable and strictly regulated legislative framework. Consequently it is IVF and embryo research – and debate over their derivative applications such as cloning, stem cell research, human admixed embryos and mitochondrial donation, which have done the most to shape both public and parliamentary perceptions of controversial biotechnological research over the past 50 years.

In many respects this is both a UK pattern and one that specifically derives from the now-extensive range of interconnected clinical and experimental procedures based on the IVF platform. However, both 'the IVF effect' that has normalised a new reproductive logic of technologically assisted fertility, and the corresponding acceptance of this condition as a fact of life are undoubtedly also global phenomena. Ten million IVF babies later, and more than 50 years after the first human egg was fertilised *in vitro* in 1968 we can safely say that IVF has been a major source of social and cultural as well as biological change. The IVF platform has also been an engine of bioscientific research and innovation, enabling a vast range of new experimental lines of enquiry from stem cell research, cloning and regenerative medicine to organoids, chimeras and *in vitro*-derived gametes. In scientific labs as well as popular culture, IVF has become part of the everyday landscape, for which the now ubiquitous image of microinjection is a familiar shorthand. In a nutshell, IVF has become an ordinary fact of life – the true measure of successful translation. For this and other reasons, we can describe IVF as one of the most successful, consequential and transformative translational technologies of our time.

All of these forces are important scientifically, in terms of how we understand and evaluate basic biological processes – such as reproduction, development and inheritance – but also how we integrate such knowledge into policy, regulation and governance. They are also important in popular culture and in everyday 'lay' models of biological (and genetic) cause and effect. Perhaps never before have the co-organisation of society and biology, economics and ecology, politics and physiology, or human rights and reproduction been so explicitly and visibly intertwined. Many of today's most important social movements across the globe are focussed on exactly these concerns (Franklin and Inhorn 2025). Struggles for racial, economic, reproductive and environmental justice are increasingly inseparable. Indigenous concerns about forests, rivers and the food chain that received little airtime twenty years ago have become not only increasingly mainstream, but are more likely to have become official government policy in many countries around the world. Maternal and child health, long a map of economic stratification and social inequality, is now a frontline issue in the promotion of new ways of thinking about long term sustainability, resilience, stability and prosperity. Similarly, new approaches to promoting and protecting global public health in the wake of COVID are ratcheting the issue of public trust in science, governments and healthcare systems higher up the scale of economic and political as well as medical importance.

All of this has implications for the relationship of science and society, and especially the maintenance of public trust – which we know from previous experience with issues such as genetically modified (GM) foods can quickly be lost – in particular when deceit, secrecy or profiteering are seen to compromise the integrity of science. It is consequently vital that the many important lessons that have been learned about building trust through public dialogue, engagement and openness are kept close at hand in the coming decades, during which better science driving better solutions will be at a premium in the face of multiple intersecting challenges. There is increasing evidence, at least for now, that the 'IVF effect' has helped to increase public trust and confidence in a more radical role for technology in the creation of new human life – especially in the UK (Franklin 2019, 2022). What is known as the 'Warnock Consensus' is but one example of the trust-dividend generated by 30 years of strict-but-permissive regulation of human fertilisation and embryology that uniquely characterises the British biotranslational landscape (Jasanoff and Metzler 2020). Given that trust is a reciprocal value, however, an area of understandable concern for many is that IVF success rates remain disappointing low, and roughly half the consumers of costly IVF services worldwide fail in their pursuit of a successful pregnancy. This trend alongside the increase in what are known as 'IVF add-ons' (extra services to help improve IVF outcomes – many of which are of unproven efficacy) coupled to the increasing commercialisation and financialisation of the fertility sector (as venture capital and large conglomerates play an increasing role in for-profit services) raise new risks for public trust such as conflicts of interest, overselling, misinformation and profiteering. These could significantly endanger the generally positive association with IVF that appears, at least for now, to bolster public confidence in experimental work with human embryos as well as the field of regenerative science more widely.

We have subtitled our book 'a sociology of biomedical translation' to foreground these key questions about how the biotranslational future will be socially shaped. As noted at the outset, this book addresses a specific question – about the history and the future of the 14 day limit – but one that encapsulates much wider issues. These not only include what lessons might be learned from reviewing the legal and scientific origins of one of the most influential pieces of translational bioscientific policy to be forged in the last half century. They also include what it means to understand bioscientific translation from a more interdisciplinary point of view, and what methodologies and concepts might help us move further in that direction. After all, if there is one stand-out lesson from the unusual history of legislating 'human fertilisation and embryology', it is undoubtedly that these are issues which affect us all.

Notes

1 The HFEA is an arm's-length public body of the Department of Health and Social Care, responsible for inspecting, licensing and monitoring fertility treatment and embryo research in the UK.
2 It is a criminal offence to keep or use embryos without a licence from the HFEA, and under section 3(3)(a) of the Act, 'a licence cannot authorise keeping or using an embryo after the appearance of the primitive streak', which is, under section 3(4), 'taken to have appeared in an embryo not later than the end of the period of 14 days beginning with the day on which the process of creating the embryo began'.
3 Michael Mulkay's comprehensive 1997 book on the embryo research debate in the UK also explores this history, and see further in Franklin (1990, 1993, 1997, 2019) and Gunning and English (1993).
4 Although it is now seldom used in practice, Schedule 2(3)(2) of the HFE Act permits 'mixing [human] sperm with the egg of a hamster, or other animal specified in Directions, for the purpose of developing more effective techniques for determining the fertility or normality of sperm, but only where anything which forms is destroyed when the research is complete and, in any event, no later than the two cell stage'.
5 Will Kymlicka (1993) has argued that Warnock prioritised agreement on conclusions over agreement on principles. Quoted in Lockwood (1988), Mary Warnock explained, 'Every sentence had to be argued over. To reach agreement on conclusions was difficult enough. To have arrived at an agreed line of argument would have been impossible.'
6 See, for example, Theodosiou and Johnson (2011) and McMillan (2021).

References

Ball, Philip (2023) '2022 Wilkins–Bernal–Medawar Lecture: Remaking Ourselves – technologies of flesh and the futures of selfhood' *Notes and Records: The Royal Society Journal of the History of Science.*

Braude, Peter (2009) 'Learning from history: the clinician's view' in Geoff Watts (ed.) *Hype, hope and hybrids: science, policy and media perspectives of the Human Fertilisation and Embryology Bill* (The Academy of Medical Sciences).

Deglincerti A. et al. (2016) 'Self-organization of the *in vitro* attached human embryo' *Nature* 533: 251–4.

Foreman, Amy L. et al. (2023) 'Human embryo models: the importance of national policy and governance review' *Current Opinion in Genetics & Development* 82: 102103.

Franklin, Sarah (1990) 'Deconstructing "desperateness": the social construction of infertility in popular media representations' in Maureen McNeil, Ian Varcoe, and Steven Yearley (eds) The new reproductive technologies (Macmillan).

Franklin, Sarah (1993) 'Making representations: the parliamentary debate on the Human Fertilisation and Embryology Act' in J. Edwards et al. *Technologies of procreation: kinship in the age of assisted conception* (Manchester University Press).

Franklin, Sarah (1997) *Embodied progress: a cultural account of assisted conception* (Routledge).

Franklin, Sarah (2013a) Biological relatives: IVF, stem cells, and the future of kinship (Duke University Press).

Franklin, Sarah (2013b) 'Conception through a looking glass: the paradox of IVF' *Reproductive BioMedicine Online* 27: 747–755.

Franklin, Sarah (2013c). 'Embryo watching: how IVF has remade biology' *TECNOSCIENZA: Italian Journal of Science & Technology Studies* 4(1): 23–44.

Franklin, Sarah (2019) 'Developmental landmarks and the Warnock Report: a sociological account of biological translation' *Comparative Studies in Society and History* 61(4): 743–773.

Franklin, Sarah (2022) *Embodied progress: a cultural account of assisted reproduction*, 2nd edition (Routledge).

Franklin, Sarah, and Inhorn, Marcia C. (eds) (2025) *The new reproductive order: changing in-fertilities around the globe* (New York University Press).

Golchin Ali et al. (2021) 'Embryonic stem cells in clinical trials: current overview of developments and challenges' *Advances in Experimental Medicine and Biology* 1312: 19–37.

Gunning, Jennifer and English, Veronica (1993) Human *in vitro* fertilization: a case study in the regulation of medical innovation (Routledge).

Hengstschläger, Markus and Rosner, Margit (2021) 'Embryoid research calls for reassessment of legal regulations' *Stem Cell Research and Therapy* 12: 356.

International Society for Stem Cell Research (2021) 'Guidelines for stem cell research and clinical translation', retrieved from www.isscr.org/policy/guidelines-for-stem-cell-research-and-clinical-translation.

Jasanoff, Sheila and Metzler, Ingrid (2020) 'Borderlands of life: IVF embryos and the law in the United States, United Kingdom and Germany' *Science, Technology and Human Values* 43(1): 1001–1037.

Kymlicka, Will (1993) 'Moral philosophy and public policy: the case of NRTs' *Bioethics* 7: 1–26.

Lockwood, Michael (1988) 'Warnock versus Powell (and Harradine): when does potentiality count?' *Bioethics* 2: 187–213.

Matthews, Kirstin R.W. and Moralí, Daniel (2020) 'National human embryo and embryoid research policies: a survey of 22 top research-intensive countries' *Regenerative Medicine* 15(7): 1905–1917.

McMillan, Catriona A.W. (2021) *The human embryo in vitro: breaking the legal stalemate* (Cambridge University Press).

Mulkay, Michael (1997) *The embryo research debate: science and the politics of reproduction* (Cambridge University Press).

Royal Society (2008) *Human Fertilisation and Embryology Bill* (Royal Society).

Shahbazi, M.N. et al. (2017) 'Self-organization of the human embryo in the absence of maternal tissues' *Nature Cell Biology* 18: 700–708.

Strathern, Marilyn (1992a) *Reproducing the future: essays on anthropology, kinship and the new reproductive technologies* (Manchester University Press).

Strathern, Marilyn (1992b) *After nature: English kinship in the late twentieth century* (Cambridge University Press)

Theodosiou, Anastasia A. and Johnson, Martin H. (2021) 'The politics of human embryo research and the motivation to achieve PGD' *Reproductive BioMedicine Online* 22: 457–471.

Warnock, Mary (1985) *A question of life: the Warnock Report on human fertilisation and embryology* (Basil Blackwell).

Parliamentary Debates

HL Deb (13 September 2018) vol. 792 col. 2440.

2 Science as a Social Contract

As we can see from the preceding observations about the intertwined sociological, biological and technological implications of IVF and embryo research, we need several different overlapping but distinct models of translation to develop effective science policy. We also need conversations that bring different disciplines together, and these are happily becoming much more common. In the realms of science policy as well as innovation, better listening has replaced more didactic approaches to the relationship of science to its many publics. This move away from a view of the public as lacking adequate knowledge or training to understand complex scientific research, and toward a practice of encouraging more public engagement with scientific innovation is known as the shift 'from deficit to dialogue'.

These important changes in how we approach the process of biological translation are particularly relevant to the UK for two main reasons. First is that the UK government's increasing emphasis on public engagement with science since the 1990s has had a significant impact on how funded scientific research projects are designed, pursued, funded and evaluated. In 2000, in response to several high-profile controversies about government science policy, a House of Lords Select Committee report on 'Science and Society' powerfully advocated the importance of genuine two-way dialogue between science and its publics, in order to increase public trust in science and produce better scientific research (House of Lords 2000). Scientific research, the report argued, can't simply be left to scientists. The public needs to have an active voice in shaping scientific priorities, and their views need to be proactive in the development of scientific research agendas, not just added on like window dressing after the fact of scientific discovery or innovation. Scientists, moreover, need to be aware not only of what they don't know but also how many of their assumptions – even about highly technical subjects – are powerfully shaped by prevailing forces that might appear to have no direct connection to the topic. Just like everyone else, scientists' identities and beliefs and values – as well as their perceptions, attitudes and experiences – are profoundly socially shaped and influenced. Scientists and government alike were firmly told they needed to listen more and pronounce less.

The specific catalyst for the unusually directive and didactic *Science and Society* report was the introduction of GM foods in the 1990s without adequate public consultation – a highly misjudged move which caused enormous controversy

DOI: 10.4324/9781003294108-2

and was seen to have gravely compromised British and European science just as the Human Genome Project (HGP) was coming to fruition. The subsequent attempt by the UK government to rewrite the social contract between science and society consequently involved more than just a superficial policy response to a public outcry. Leading parliamentary and scientific bodies worked hand-in-hand with prominent academics – including sociologists, philosophers, psychologists and historians – to dig deep into the sources of acute social unrest around GM, which ultimately were seen to involve a combination of evasion, arrogance and to some degree actual deception. These very serious failures of both judgement and communication led in turn to a shift within both science policy circles and the professional scientific community that came to be known as the 'turn to dialogue'. This 'sea change' in professional scientific culture effectively reversed the way in which public engagement with science was previously viewed, transforming it from a process of 'informing' the public about the benefits scientific research into an exploration of public views, listening to them carefully, evaluating insights gained through public dialogue and then using the findings to improve translational outcomes.

Research has shown not only that the 'turn to dialogue' was very quickly and seriously adopted by (most of) the UK scientific community from 2000 onwards, but also that many scientists have come to appreciate why greater public input into scientific projects is a win-win proposition (Burchell et al. 2009). This brings us to a second important reason why the UK's research climate for innovative bioscientific research is unusually permissive while also being highly regulated, which is the powerful role of central government whose policies are enforced both through national funding agencies such as UKRI (UK Research and Innovation) and regulatory bodies such as the Health Research Authority.

'Translational' science is also a term that dates to the turn of the millennium and reflects the 'push' from science policy toward innovation that was strongly favoured by both the Blair and Clinton governments (as epitomised by the Human Genome Project). 'Translation' or the 'translational process' are terms used to describe an iterative sequence of research development from discovery to innovation, often referred to as a 'pipeline'. Traditionally, the translational pipeline begins with basic scientific research and proof of concept, leading to the next stage which is adaptation of scientific discoveries that have the potential to improve health outcomes into clinical procedures. In turn, potentially successful clinical innovations are tested and refined through clinical trials, taking them 'from bench to bedside'. The final stage in the translational process is the scaling up of clinically safe and successful procedures into widespread use and commercially profitable markets. We saw a remarkable example of rapid and successful biomedical translation in the context of COVID, as new vaccines were developed in the lab, successfully trialled and safely scaled up to mass manufacture at unprecedented speeds.

What we also saw in the context of COVID was the familiar phenomenon of suspicious publics who neither trusted nor agreed to use vaccines. As in the GM controversy in the 1990s, the role of government was widely criticised – especially in terms of how it communicated about certain risks, and also what it did not communicate about its decision-making processes to the general public. Regardless of whether the government could have acted differently, or the public's distrust was justified, these tensions confirm a crucial principle at the heart of the translational process, which is that in order for beneficial scientific discoveries to have an impact they need to be trusted by enough people for their benefits to be realised. The lower the levels of public trust in a new technology, the less it can be used for the public good.

In the same way, then, that the earlier one-way model of scientific communication with the public, known as the 'deficit model', unhelpfully positioned the 'lay' public as lacking adequate knowledge to make informed decisions about science, and therefore as 'ignorant' subjects requiring guidance from scientists about the 'correct facts', so too the one-way model of the translational pipeline – which positions public acceptance of the new technology as a taken-for-granted outcome or end-point – has given way to a dialogic, or two-way ground-up model of 'growing' or 'incubating' successful technologies, by incorporating public views much earlier in the innovation process. Today, successful translational science – just like successful basic experimental research – is seen more as an ecosystem, with many interacting forces and complex feedback loops that defy simple one-way explanations. Top-down, managerial solutions based on simplistic models of control all too often yield precisely the unexpected and undesirable outcomes they were allegedly designed to mitigate.

One of the only principles that seems to function as a consistently reliable compass on the bumpy landscape of biomedical translation is the trust effect. This is a complicated principle in part because trust is emotional as well as intellectual. People often describe trust as something they either have or are willing to extend, and it is also described, like respect, as something that can be won or lost. Trust may or may not take time to earn, but it can be lost more or less instantaneously. Moreover, the sudden loss of hard-earned trust can not only have a huge impact in itself, but can generate significant and lasting consequences, including an aftermath (or afterburn) of betrayal, anger, grief, disbelief and alienation. One of the most common words for loss of trust is 'violate', and another is 'breach'.

Conversely, one of the ways in which trust is strengthened is through being tested and re-confirmed. One of the most familiar sources of trust is simply the passage of time: 'tried and tested' is another way to describe a method or relationship that is considered safe, reliable and trustworthy. The philosopher Onora O'Neill similarly points to the essential link between trust, accountability and trustworthiness: trust is strengthened by the ability to evaluate claims as trustworthy through repeated verification. Indeed, where such evaluation is not needed – for example when facts and outcomes are clearly known, trust is not required. Trust is needed when there is risk, and thus by definition, as O'Neill puts it, 'trust must run ahead of proof or control … [It] is redundant where I [already] have effective guarantees' (O'Neill 2014: 179). This is why trust is so important both to the relationship between science and its publics, and to biomedical translation.

A final important point thus concerns the relationships between trust and uncertainty, and trust and opposition. While much research confirms that high levels of uncertainty about scientific outcomes or medical risks are associated with lower levels of trust, research has also shown that the key variable is not always the presence of verifiable, or trustworthy, knowledge – but instead the source of information combined with how uncertainties and risks are communicated. How people evaluate risks also depends crucially on what is at stake. Research in the context of uncertainty around prenatal genetic testing, for example, counter-intuitively suggests that explicit disclosure of uncertainty, and candid – or even exaggerated – accounts of risk, may increase patients' trust in new and controversial technologies, due to the greater confidence they gain in the integrity and reliability of the information they are being given. So called 'positive effects of uncertainty communication' have been shown to be particularly significant in health contexts, where the ratio of what is at stake to what can be known may be low, but the source of information (i.e. health professionals) is highly trusted (Steijaert et al. 2021). This finding is not so surprising when we consider the opposite scenario – of over-confident reassurances decreasing trust in their source, and also when we think of different contexts, such the airline industry or food standards authority, where high levels of uncertainty would be less likely to engender confidence. The turn to dialogue in UK science was explicitly aimed to rebuild trust not only through increased communication, openness and transparency, but also by establishing a long-term culture change through which professional science would become both more responsive to and more engaged with the general public, better at openly expressing uncertainty, and thus better at building and retaining trust (Burchell et al. 2009).

Reciprocity and Public Trust

The National Health Service (NHS) is a third feature which has helped to establish the UK's unusually stable, permissive and supportive climate for innovative biomedical translation. Since its inception in 1948, the NHS has been viewed as a 'National Treasure' emblematising core values of Britishness such as decency, generosity, and care for the most vulnerable in society. The NHS is both loved and trusted due to its commitment to equality of provision and fairness – offering a safety net for all who need it regardless of their circumstances. These ideals may never have been fully met through the NHS, and these values are not shared by every British citizen, but the NHS is nonetheless the embodiment not only of a practical objective but a national ideal. As the highly respected British social policy theorist Richard Titmuss famously argued in 1970, the NHS both expresses and confirms a set of shared ethical values, and these are affirmed as a social bond through acts of altruism such as donating blood – a literal gift of life to strangers that affirms a communal ethic of egalitarian and inclusive social welfare (Titmuss 1970).

Although much has changed in the half-century since Titmuss published his iconic analysis of its virtues, the NHS continues to stand out as one of the definitive national symbols of contemporary Britishness, and in particular Britain's distinctive value system as a society. Moreover, the core idea from Titmuss's work – that altruism, solidarity and reciprocity are the key underlying values binding citizens to the values of the NHS – still aligns well with how many British people regard their health system. In addition to the huge public appreciation for the NHS expressed during the COVID pandemic, Titmuss's model of the NHS has had something of a rebirth in the context of genomic science, which relies heavily on anonymised donation to create the essential – and very large – databases on which the translation of genomic data into useful applications crucially depends. Many policy reports on genomic medicine, for example, explicitly use Titmuss's framework in which altruism, solidarity and reciprocity form the basis of both the shared communal ethic supporting the NHS, the implicit social bonds that flow from this reciprocal system, and the benefits it brings to all (Tutton 2002, 2004).

Although Titmuss does not himself use the concept of the 'social contract' in his 1970 book, this term has frequently been used by others to connect the values of reciprocity, solidarity and altruism connected with the NHS to a more overarching idea of social belonging, and in particular the idea of exchange. Within social anthropology, systems of exchange that rely upon ceremonial gift-giving exhibit what the sociologist Marcel Mauss (1954) codified as 'the law of the gift'. This refers to the power relation inherent in gift-giving and the inevitably implied, or imposed, obligation to reciprocate, or return the gift that results from a transaction in which one person gives to another. This interpretation of gift-giving is most relevant to societies in which the giving of gifts is not only frequent and highly structured, but highly integrated with other social institutions such as kinship, clanship, succession and rituals surrounding key events such as births, deaths and harvests. To some, such as the British anthropologist Mary Douglas (1970), the highly structured nature of gift-giving within the exchange economies of pre-modern societies confirms that there is no such thing as a 'free gift'. All gifts confer obligations, in this view, and they are also part of an overarching 'grammar' of social obligation that deeply informs both explicit and implicit moral codes of conduct.

Titmuss argued, in contrast, that the altruistic spirit that is so vital to the modern NHS ensures that unpaid blood donation is indeed a 'free' gift to strangers. However, one can argue it nonetheless confers an obligation of reciprocity – albeit upon the state, rather than the recipient of the gift. Moreover, this reciprocity is in the form not only of an implied social obligation but arguably an explicit social contract in the sense that it both underwrites, and is underwritten by, the relationship between the citizen and the state (including through taxation). We might suggest, for example, that whereas the gift relation described by Mauss involves a direct dyadic relation between two parties, the Titmuss model of 'the gift relationship' is triangular, involving the giver, the receiver and the state that organises the transaction between all three parties. Crucially, however, we can also describe the tripartite Titmuss model as both 'mutual' and 'reflexive' in that the relation between the giver and the state is not so much that of the receiver and the state in reverse as the same relation on both sides, which is one of trust. Indeed, to the extent it is trust that is the most essential shared currency according to the Titmuss model, we might also conclude that the social value the NHS most powerfully articulates in the British context is a trust economy, in which altruism and reciprocity not only express solidarity but function somewhat like a bank, or mutual fund.

Titmuss's argument about blood donation was also important because by comparing the trust-based British altruistic system to the American practice of paying donors he could show that the British system was not only cheaper, more resilient and fairer – but safer. Collecting blood from people who donate because they want to significantly increases both the quality and the consistency of the blood supply, he showed, while also improving overall confidence in the healthcare system as a whole. Conversely, paying donors leads to a much higher contribution to the blood supply from people who need to sell their blood and may be more likely not to disclose key information about their health. As a result, and again somewhat counterintuitively, not paying people to donate blood saves everyone money, and even 'pays for itself' as a system, because the quality of blood is higher and the costs of contamination reduced.

Blood was a useful example for making this argument and it is a highly symbolic substance as well. Amidst the more recent short-term, shareholder-focussed and austerity-driven trends of privatisation of healthcare and social welfare services, as well as of public utilities such as water, rail and electricity, there is increasing interest in the idea of 'social purpose' economics which extends corporate responsibility, or fiscal or civic duty, to focus on the delivery of social goods as a top priority. For ethical-values-first companies such as Patagonia, this has meant literally re-incorporating as a social welfare organisation in order to devote all their future profits to combatting climate change. The wider question for other public and private companies – including Foundation-owned behemoths like IKEA, Rolex or in the UK the Cadbury or Rowntree companies – is how to deliver sustainable and competitive economic performance while also contributing to the public good. In exploring the question of trust, transparency, health, citizenship, the economy, the state and the social contracts or shared values connecting these values and institutions, it is worth returning to the question of the Warnock Consensus engendered by the 14 day rule.

From the Social Contract to the IVF Industry

While the House of Lords committee examining 'Science and Society' chaired by Roy Jenkins was wringing its hands over the 'urgent crises' of public trust in science in the late 1990s, they might instructively have cast an eye back over the UK legislative framework set up to regulate 'human fertilisation and embryology' a decade earlier. In contrast to the over-confident denials of the risks of cattle-borne prions (BSE) and GM foods, and subsequent ministerial U-turns, resignations and apologies, Mary Warnock offered a masterclass to anyone watching closely of how to handle risk, uncertainty and uncharted scientific territory with great success. In lieu of the legal vacuum she was tasked to fill, Warnock left a full docket for the press, parliamentarians and the public to ponder over – as well as a comprehensive set of briefing papers containing numerous concrete proposals. As we shall see in Chapter 3, the Warnock approach to the complete unknown was to provide not one but several different maps, and to establish landmarks as well as well-lit paths to guide people through the legal *terra nullius* of 'human fertilisation and embryology'. She also ran her committee much like a classroom, providing an extensive curriculum made up of briefing papers, expert testimony and communications from a huge range of interested parties, all shepherded into clear agendas, diagrams and objectives for every meeting.

After she and her Committee had submitted their Report in 1984, and presented it to Parliament, as well as the public and the press, Mary Warnock and Anne McLaren toured the country and travelled abroad to make the case for their proposed legislative infrastructure. As we explore further in Chapter 3, they faced complete rejection and incomprehension in some quarters and apathy in others, but above all and from the start they faced intensive opposition to both embryo research and IVF as well as to surrogacy, gamete donation and artificial insemination from within Parliament as well as the media, general public and religious authorities. Their approach was to engage with as many and as wide a range of viewpoints as possible – McLaren even travelling to Rome to lobby the Pope on the need for IVF and embryo research. Undaunted by counterarguments from friends as well as foes, they relied on the sound underlying logic of the proposed Human Fertilisation and Embryology Bill and Licensing Authority, which would oversee a Code of Practice backed by the will of Parliament and enforced, if necessary, through criminal law. Their logic, at root, was that IVF and embryo research would help people and be good for society, but that they had to be sensibly and credibly regulated in order to maintain public confidence and trust.

Engaging directly with their audience, delivering the arguments, presenting the evidence and outlining a clear path forward were the means by which Warnock and McLaren sought to gain the trust of professionals, legislators, the press, the public and the government. Rather than avoiding discussions about the inherent uncertainties and risks implicit in a new scientific field, or the doubts shared by many people (including many scientists) concerning the future of test-tube baby science, they met these inevitable questions head on in the confidence that they had good arguments to persuade people to support their proposals for well-regulated research into human fertilisation and embryology. They succeeded in the end because a majority of the members of all of the opposing constituencies eventually agreed with them. The Warnock Report explicitly recognised that embryo research and IVF treatment exist on a continuum and are interdependent. Without research on human embryos, IVF would not exist as a treatment for infertility, and without IVF it would not be possible to study the earliest stages of human development *in vitro*. This was a crucial point because supporting IVF without allowing embryo research would impose a huge price on the very community to whom the 'miracle baby' technique was intended to offer precious new hope. As Peter Braude and Martin Johnson (1989) explained, if IVF continued without ongoing embryo research, women would become its experimental subjects:

Instead of conducting research on small groups of living cells in culture it will be the women seeking treatment by these means who will themselves become the subjects of the experiment.

(Braude and Johnson 1989: 1350)

Moreover, this point is not complex: IVF has a punishingly high failure rate, and it is women and couples who are already suffering the consequences of unwanted childlessness who pay the highest price for yet another round of disappointment. Although success rates have improved significantly since the mid-1980s, the most likely outcome for every cycle of IVF continues to be failure: in 2021, the birth rate per embryo transferred for women under the age of 35 was 33 per cent (HFEA 2023a). Research on human embryos continues to be needed in order to further refine the techniques of IVF and make it more likely to succeed. As the Warnock Report (1984) put it, this fact is 'essential' to the future of infertility treatment:

> We do not want to see a situation in which human embryos are frivolously or unnecessarily used in research but we are bound to take account of the fact that the advances in the treatment of infertility, which we have discussed in the earlier part of this report, could not have taken place without such research; and that continued research is essential, if advances in treatment and medical knowledge are to continue.
>
> (Warnock 1984: para 11.18)

In addition to the fact that embryo research is a necessary prerequisite for IVF, another way in which embryo research and IVF exist on a continuum is that the vast majority of embryos used in research started their life in an IVF clinic. Almost all research embryos were created so that they would be available for use in a patient's treatment. If some embryos are judged to be non-viable or otherwise unsuitable for use in treatment, and therefore also unsuitable for freezing for future use, the patient (and her partner, if she has one) will need to decide whether to discard them or donate them to research. If the patient has frozen embryos in storage after she has completed her family, once again, she (and her partner) have a decision to make. They could donate their unwanted frozen embryos for use in another patient's treatment, or they could allow them to perish, or they could donate them for use in research or training.

The inflexibility of the current law – which hampers opportunities for donation, by requiring that embryos are donated to a specific project of research, rather than to an embryo 'bank' – is at odds with consistently high levels of patient willingness to donate embryos for research purposes. In a study of factors affecting patient perceptions of embryo donation to stem cell research at Guy's and St Thomas's Centre for PGD, Franklin et al. (2005) found that 67 per cent of patients were willing to donate their embryos for use in research, of whom more than 80 per cent said that they wanted to 'give something back'. It is also common for patients to say that it would be wasteful to discard embryos which could be put to good use in a research project (Franklin et al. 2005; Lyerly et al. 2006). Although donating embryos for use in the treatment of others would also put those embryos to good use, it is a decision which undoubtedly comes with more emotional 'baggage', because it may mean being contacted in the future by any resulting children, who will be one's own children's genetic siblings.

Indeed, it could be argued that the donation of embryos by IVF patients for use in research is a particularly potent example of Titmuss's 'two-way' reciprocal model of the public good (Franklin 2006). Once patients have given consent to their embryos' use in research, the embryos move from clinic to laboratory, and there will be times when the benefits of that research then flow back to the clinic, in order to improve outcomes for future IVF patients. Even when the gains from basic research may be less direct and immediate, patients in general benefit from receiving treatment within an environment which values scientific research.

As sociologist Richard Tutton (2002) has explained, Titmuss's model of the gift relationship emphasises the expressive, meaningful and symbolic dimensions of its social importance as well as its practical advantages. As Tutton notes, the idea of 'giving something back' has achieved 'metaphorical resonance as part of a broader political discourse on the values of social equality, altruism and community', and should consequently be recognised as 'essentially a political conceptualization of the British donor system, defending the welfare state, and attacking the commercialism represented by the US system of market-based healthcare'. But if the donation of embryos to research by IVF patients is an example of the sort of altruistic two-way social contract which is emblematic of the UK welfare state, and in particular of the NHS, how might this be affected by the increasing commercialisation of IVF and the fertility industry?

When the Warnock Report was published in 1984, there were few providers of fertility treatment, and lengthy waiting lists (para 2.17). The Warnock Report recommended more provision of fertility treatment within the NHS, and the setting up of a working group 'to consider how best an IVF service can be organised within the NHS' (para 5.11). It recognised that there would be 'private IVF clinics alongside those within the NHS', but the Committee 'believe[d] it is important that there should be a sufficient level of NHS provision for childless couples not to feel that their only recourse is to the private sector' (para 5.11). This has never happened.

Even though the Warnock Report acknowledged that private clinics would continue to coexist with NHS treatment services, it did not foresee the emergence of such a large and lucrative market in private fertility treatment. As a result, the Human Fertilisation and Embryology Act 1990 does not give the HFEA the sort of powers it might need in order to regulate a flourishing commercial market. The HFEA cannot control the prices that clinics charge, and it has limited powers over the marketing of unregulated 'add on' services,[1] even where there is zero evidence of their efficacy in improving success rates (Cirkovic et al. 2023).

In 2023, the UK fertility industry was worth £627 million, and it grew by 4.4 per cent in 2022, considerably faster than the rest of the economy (IBIS World 2023). In the past, private clinics were typically set up and run by doctors who specialised in the treatment of infertility. Now it is increasingly common for clinics to have merged into very large conglomerates, and for venture capital to fund and sell on start-up companies. Sociologist Lucy van de Wiel (2020) has described how egg freezing, in particular, has attracted considerable investment from private equity and venture capital, as investors have recognised its potential to expand the market for fertility services beyond people who are currently struggling to conceive.

Increases in the age of first-time mothers, and the legalisation of same sex marriage are also seen as growth opportunities for the fertility sector.

New start-ups not only offer treatment services, but also financial products, such as 'fertility insurance' policies for employees (van der Wiel 2020). In addition to extending the market for fertility services by selling treatments such as egg freezing to young, presumed-to-be-fertile women, another way to expand the fertility industry's customer base is to offer consumer credit options, so that patients can undergo private treatment despite being unable to afford them. Although facilitating the debt-financing of IVF treatments that are beyond their means to people who can't otherwise afford to pay for them may well widen access to such services, there are inevitable conflicts of interest if doctors are recommending treatments to patients at the same time as offering them a credit facility to pay for them. Moreover, since IVF fails in roughly two-thirds of cycles, 'lenders might be more interested in financing successive rounds of treatment (at potentially successively higher rates of interest)' (Jacoby 2009). For lenders, patients who have suffered repeated IVF failure, or whose treatment is otherwise very unlikely to succeed, are a lucrative source of revenue, and this may be at odds with clinicians' duty of care to offer frank advice about the wisdom of continued treatment.

But if the IVF industry has become more transactional and profit-driven, this is less true of the basic scientific research, often involving donated human embryos, that is essential for improving IVF success rates and validating new IVF add-ons such as aneuploidy testing. Research on human embryos, and for that matter into human reproductive and developmental biology more generally, is largely undertaken either in, or in close partnership with, publicly funded laboratories. In the UK such research is largely undertaken by publicly funded scientists, and is highly dependent on patients who are willing to donate their embryos – many of whom report being motivated by reciprocity and altruism. Whereas the IVF industry, in other words, is clearly moving in a more commercial direction, the embryo research on which it depends not only remains largely within, but in many ways classically epitomises, the voluntary, reciprocal, altruism-motivated gift-and-trust based economy described by Titmuss, and embodied by the NHS.

Indeed, compared to other contexts of donation, the literature on embryo donation shows a high and consistent level of trust in health professionals and strongly positive attitudes towards medical research. In their systematic review of more than a decade of such research, including both qualitative and quantitative research on embryo disposition decision-making, Samorinha and colleagues found that:

> those who donate embryos for research reported feelings of reciprocity towards science and medicine, revealed a positive vision of research and high levels of trust in the medical system. Additionally, they described such a decision as an opportunity to help others, by contributing to a healthier world and to the improvement of IVF treatments.
>
> (Samorinha et al. 2014)

It has never been seriously suggested that patients should be paid for the embryos they give to research. Through donation, the status of stored embryos shifts from potential offspring/sibling to biological material, but not – crucially – to private property which could be bought and sold. But even if patients who have paid thousands of pounds for a cycle of IVF nevertheless express a desire to 'give something back' by donating their unused embryos to research, in practice, comparatively few are given this option. As the Progress Educational Trust argued in its response to the HFEA's consultation on modernising the HFEA Act:

> Under the present regime, scandalously large numbers of unused human embryos go to waste in the UK – often without patients ever being given the option to donate embryos to research, and sometimes in direct contravention of their wishes … [W]e have heard accounts of patients wishing to donate unused embryos, who have taken it upon themselves to track down and contact relevant researchers – only to discover that they are unable to donate their embryos, for legal or practical reasons.
>
> (Progress Educational Trust 2023)

This situation – reflecting a growing disconnect between the commercial ethos of the fertility industry and the gift economy on which embryo research depends – raises a number of important practical, moral, regulatory and sociological questions that would repay further research. There is clearly a tension here that could undermine trust in government and health policy as well as science and in particular the future of embryo research in potentially controversial areas such as embryo modelling. For our purposes here, it is important to point out that the future of the 14 day rule is also implicated in this set of tensions and questions. In so far as the 14 day rule is both an explicit regulatory policy but also a social contract, according to which the human embryo research is permitted subject to both strict oversight and a legal limit of 14 days, it is also, we have argued, an expressive piece of legislation that symbolises as well as enacts all of these principles – and has done so for a substantial period of time.

Conclusion

So far we have argued that the 14 day limit and its translation into law and guidance in many very different jurisdictions represents a pivotal achievement in terms not only of policy but translation. Both the 14 day limit, and the principles on which is was based, enabled the Warnock Committee to persuade an often sceptical public, as well as adamantly opposed parliamentarians, to accept a workable and enforceable framework for the regulation of embryo research which was enacted in 1990 and has stood the test of time for more than three decades. The resulting Warnock Consensus has enabled a high degree of public trust to support innovative translational research, and this unusually level of support is rightly seen to demonstrate the value of *beneficial limits* for science and scientists, as well as for society more generally. In taking seriously the concerns of the public, and setting reassuring red lines around what can be done to human embryos, the 14 day rule embodies the social contract or exchange model of scientific research advocated by Titmuss and widely seen to be at the heart of the NHS.

As the first steps in the UK are taken towards a review of the Human Fertilisation and Embryology Act 1990 (HFEA 2023b), with the prospect of new reforming legislation within the next few years, it is worth reflecting on what aspects of the existing statutory scheme need to be preserved, as well as focussing on the need for reform. Our contention in this book is that the 14 day limit has a value beyond setting a numerical time limit for research on human embryos. Instead, it embodies an approach to the regulation of research which 'care[s] for new forms of human life by building collective common sense and publicly sanctioned moral reasoning' (Jasanoff and Metzler 2020). This careful approach to regulation has resulted in what might be described as an unusually conducive climate for embryo research in the UK, which, as Baroness Bottomley put it in the House of Lords, should not be taken for granted.

> The fact that it has now become a relatively quiet issue does not mean that it does not have the potential to become once again extremely noisy. It speaks for the hugely effective way in which the HFEA has gone about its work, and the confidence that it has built not only in the United Kingdom among all parties but, as has rightly been said, around the world.
>
> (HL Deb 9 May 2011)

At some point in the future, the 14 day limit may be replaced by a different and most likely an extended time limit, but the existence of a line (or lines) beyond which scientists must not go, will nevertheless continue to be a crucial feature of the regulation of embryo research. It may also be that given the very large range of entities that now fall under the category of 'embryoid' that other demarcations are needed, and these might include categories of permitted and impermissible use, or genealogies or taxonomies defined by sources and origins of materials, permissible and impermissible methods, and acceptable or unacceptable purposes of research. Whichever criteria are used, the maintenance of public trust will crucially depend on findings derived from extensive public engagement and dialogue. In order to take seriously public concerns and engender public confidence and trust, it will be vital to engage in a wide-reaching dialogue about not only the relationship between IVF and embryo research, but the importance of high quality scientific research to reproductive healthcare and fertility equity more widely. It will be essential too that scientists, regulators and other key experts participate in the communication and dialogue process in order that robust findings from such exercises can be integrated into the development of both research objectives and science policy. We would add that the social values and benefits associated with human embryo, egg and gamete donation for research need to continue to be investigated and incorporated into the analysis of public attitudes toward and perceptions of new areas of research such as embryo modelling.[2] We would also advise that careful consideration is given to the potential for public trust in both research and policy in the sensitive area of human fertilisation and embryology to be undermined by excessive commercialisation of fertility services including the marketing of IVF, egg freezing and contested 'add-ons' such as aneuploidy testing.

Finally, our analysis of the 'lessons learned' from history of the 14 day rule over the past three decades suggests that whatever permissions are allowed in the future need to conform to two key criteria: (1) they must be conditional on agreed limits that are clear, unambiguous, enforceable and credible; and (2) there must be mechanisms both within and outside the scientific community to ensure the permissible limits are robustly maintained, with adequate sanctions in place to ensure compliance. These 2 provisions are not only needed to reassure the public and government as well as legislators: they are also essential to promoting the future of excellence in scientific research. As we shall see in the next two chapters, the science the 14 day rule is designed to promote is deeply intertwined with the fascinating story of how, exactly, these principles were implemented by the Warnock Committee and together they continue to offer a textbook example of how best to promote public trust at the same time as protecting basic science.

Notes

1 The HFEA's statutory remit is the regulation of human *fertilisation* and embryology, which means that some treatments 'for infertility' lie outside of its powers.
2 It may be, for example, that the understandably comprehensive and extensive consent process designed for use at the very outset of human embryonic cell line derivation and banking no longer needs to remain as detailed, and that requirements such as the need to specify the precise uses of all donated embryos donated to research is no longer necessary – especially if it is now posing and impediment to such donations.

References

Braude, Peter and Johnson, Martin (1989) 'Embryo research: yes or no?' *British Medical Journal* 299: 1349.

Burchell, Kevin, Franklin, Sarah and Holden, Kerry (2009) *Public culture as professional science: final report of the ScoPE project* (BIOS).

Cirkovic, Stevan et al. (2023) 'Is the use of IVF add-on treatments driven by patients or clinics? Findings from a UK patient survey' *Human Fertility* 26(2): 365–372.

Douglas, Mary (1970) *Natural symbols* (Barrie and Rockliff).

Franklin, Sarah et al. (2005) 'Factors affecting PGD patients' consent to donate embryos to stem cell research' paper presented at the Sixth International Symposium on Preimplantation Genetics, London, 19–21 May (see conference programme and abstracts, *Reproductive BioMedicine Online* 10(Suppl. 2): 31).

Franklin, Sarah (2006) 'Embryonic economies: the double reproductive value of stem cells' *BioSocieties* 1(1): 71–90.

HFEA (2023a) *Fertility treatment 2021: preliminary trends and figures* (HFEA).

HFEA (2023b) *Modernising the regulation of fertility treatment and research involving human embryos* (HFEA).

House of Lords (2000) *Science and society* (HMSO).

IBIS World (2023) 'Fertility clinics in the UK – market size 2011–2029' retrieved from www.ibisworld.com/united-kingdom/market-size/fertility-clinics.

Jacoby, Melissa B. (2009) 'The debt financing of parenthood' *Law and Contemporary Problems* 72(3): 147–175.

Jasanoff, Sheila and Metzler, Ingrid (2020) 'Borderlands of life: IVF embryos and the law in the United States, United Kingdom and Germany' *Science, Technology and Human Values* 43(1): 1001–1037.

Lyerly, Anne Drapkin et al. (2006) 'Factors that affect infertility patients' decisions about disposition of frozen embryos' *Fertility and Sterility* 85(6): 1623–1630.

Mauss, Marcel (1954) *The gift: forms and functions of exchange in archaic societies* (Cohen and West).

O'Neill, Onora (2014) 'Trust, trustworthiness, and accountability' in Nicholas Morris and David Vines (eds) *Capital failure: Rebuilding trust in financial services* (Oxford University Press) 172–189.

Progress Educational Trust (2023) *Modernising the regulation of fertility treatment and research involving human embryos: consultation response by PET* 14 April (Progress Educational Trust).

Samorinha, Catarina, Pereira, Margarida, Machado, Helena, Figueiredo, Bárbara and Silva, Susana (2014) 'Factors associated with the donation and non-donation of embryos for research: a systematic review' Human Reproduction Update 20(5): 641–655.

Steijaert, Mickey J., Schaap, Gabi and Riet, Jonathan Van't (2021) 'Two-sided science: communicating scientific uncertainty increases trust in scientists and donation intention by decreasing attribution of communicator bias' *Communications* 46: 297–316.

Titmuss, Richard (1970) *The gift relationship: from human blood to social policy* (Allen & Unwin).

Tutton, Richard (2002) 'Gift relationships in genetics research' *Science as Culture* 11(4): 523–542.

Tutton, Richard (2004) 'Person, property and gift' in Oonagh Corrigan and Richard Tutton (eds) *Genetic databases: socio-ethical issues in the collection and use of DNA* (Routledge): 19–39.

Van de Wiel, Lucy (2020) 'The speculative turn in IVF: egg freezing and the financialization of fertility' *New Genetics and Society* 39(3): 306–326.

Warnock Committee (1984) *Report of the Committee of Enquiry into Human Fertilisation and Embryology* (HMSO).

Parliamentary Debates

HL Deb (9 May 2011) vol. 727 col. 686.

3 The Scientific Origins of the 14 Day Rule

When it was founded in 1948, the NHS was widely understood as a gift to the nation in return for the huge sacrifices of the population during World War II (Hart 2010). The new health service, along with state-sponsored social support systems that provided a safety net for all, were accompanied by new educational and employment opportunities that rapidly expanded in the 1950s. The baby-boom that followed not only marked a generational shift, but ushered in one of the longest periods of sustained economic growth in British history. This period also saw enormous growth in the biological sciences, and it was in the early 1950s that an American and several British scientists unravelled the physical structure of DNA – the famous double helix – confirmed in the Cavendish Laboratory on Free School Lane in Cambridge on 28 February 1953. Transforming the aftermath of war into the gift of universal healthcare was part of the new social – and socialist – contract that linked the NHS to both major government investments into medical and scientific research facilities and a new view of experimental science as a public good and shared resource.

The interest in genetics that brought an American scientist funded by the US Atomic Energy Commission to a Cambridge physics laboratory was a direct expression of this significant translational watershed. As the distinguished feminist historian of science and physicist, Evelyn Fox Keller (2003) has noted, the huge transfer of resources into the life sciences in the wake of two world wars was not only a literal transformation of swords into ploughshares (and new crops), but a change in mindset – marking a newly explicit commitment by government to promote and celebrate science for its many publics, and to increase the role of the state in the funding of large-scale science projects as well as scientific training. The primary goal of new organisations such as the National Science Foundation in the United States as well as the NHS in Britain was to enhance prosperity by investing in research that would deliver better health, more efficient food production, and revolutionary research into the basic building blocks of life itself. It was no coincidence it was in a lab directed by Ernest Rutherford, the physicist who split the atom, that Watson and Crick cracked open DNA. Radiation linked these two experiments through its transformative effects on elementary particles, but also fundamentally divided them as atomic weapons gave way to a new war on disease.

DOI: 10.4324/9781003294108-3

Biological control – or getting a better handle on biology – was one of the chief scientific objectives influencing the evolution of the life sciences in the mid-twentieth century, and genes played an increasingly headline role in this process. From its inception, the study of genetics – be it in mammals, plants or micro-organisms – has always been concerned with the interplay between the mechanisms of biological conservation and transmutation – the magic paradox of how all living organisms 'know' how to stay the same but also change and evolve. Intriguingly, but perplexingly, these opposing forces are always co-present and intimately intertwined but also clearly separate: a fish does not become a squirrel (until it does). Even within the context of a single chromosome, genes move, 'jump', break and transpose – remaking themselves to both 'hold the line', but also swerve. Sexual reproduction vastly complicates the process of tracking genetic change by enabling the wholescale recombination of the genomes of two individuals. This has always been the mystery of genetic expression, and intergenerational transmission, and it is also why the study of the relationships between reproduction, developmental biology and inheritance is one of the most ambitious and compelling arenas of biological calculus.

The 1950s was a key period in the development of tools to study these relations, and as we investigate the origins of the 14 day rule it is worth pausing to consider some of the technical challenges involved in this area of study, as well as some of the key British scientists involved in it, not least because it was not anticipated mid-century that one of the key tools for unravelling the complexity of genetic expression within and between cells would be IVF. Indeed, in the same way it was not anticipated even in the 1980s that IVF would become a major clinical technology, or that within less than four decades an IVF baby would be born every 45 seconds, the research implications of the IVF platform for basic biological research had only barely begun to be envisaged as late as the 1990s and were not widely appreciated until the post-millennial dawn of the the IVF-stem cell interface (Franklin 2013) brought them more clearly into view.

A small but significant exception to the slow awakening to IVF's research importance was the mammalian developmental biology community – a particularly strong group in the UK, with major research centres in Oxford, Cambridge, London and Edinburgh throughout the twentieth century – and a string of major discoveries in its latter half that have dramatically reshaped the landscape of translational science in this century. Unsurprisingly, since both IVF and embryo transfer were both invented and perfected in the labs of reproductive and developmental biologists, who initially used it as an experimental research technique in basic bench science, the view from the IVF window had a small but avid audience among mid-twentieth century researchers seeking to understand the intimate mechanics of human fertilisation and embryology, and in particular how they were connected to inheritance.

One of the most important scientists who helped refine the use of IVF as a research tool as early as the 1950s was Dr Anne McLaren, who later became the chief architect of the 14 day rule alongside Mary Warnock. McLaren's famous self-description was that she was interested in studying 'everything involved in getting from one generation to the next'. Like her progressively minded contemporary Richard Titmuss, McLaren was deeply concerned with social justice and welfare as well as biological science. Also like Titmuss, she understood human fertility to be both a social and biological condition, and a crucial component of human social, economic and political life. The first woman in her family to go to university, despite (or perhaps because of) her aristocratic upbringing, McLaren went on to become one of the most acclaimed scientists in her field and of her generation, while also becoming increasingly involved in the politics of science, scientific ethics and science policy. She became the first woman to hold office in the Royal Society, as its Foreign Secretary (1991–1996), and took a leading role in many international scientific organisations as well as serving as an advisor to innumerable advisory committees, governments and regulatory bodies.

From the very start of her research career in the 1950s, McLaren sought to unravel some of the most difficult and challenging questions concerning the precise biological mechanisms guiding the very earliest critical events in mammalian development – an almost impossible topic to study given the dearth of available tools, equipment, and procedures needed for such work. As well as the lack of precedent in terms of experimental methods, equipment and laboratory infrastructure to support elementary research into mammalian embryology and reproductive physiology, such investigations were notoriously difficult. Credible findings required more than individual studies: they needed a degree of scale to be conclusive. In turn, scaling up required extensive standardisation, repetition and duplication: to establish the necessary controls and confirm the reliability of the results the whole experimental system had to support hundreds and even thousands of precise procedures – all rigorously timed and coordinated as part of a systematic, cyclical, no-stone-left-unturned experimental design. The mammalian development community was small and tight knit in no small part due to these daunting entry requirements.

Fascinated by the reproductive process, and in particular the complexity of the interaction between the developing embryo and the maternal environment – and not lacking in stamina – McLaren chose a classic biological problem as one of her first major research topics, namely the question of 'maternal effect'. Long an apocryphal and familiar gestational trope, the idea of the mother's body picking up and carrying influences that shape her progeny has taken many forms, including Jacob's famous Biblical use of striped rods to create spotted sheep. A related nineteenth-century theory, of telegony – or 'sire effect' – postulated that a female animal could transmit the paternal imprint of her first pregnancy onto later offspring, in effect re-fathering them (the famous test case was of a mare who gave birth to offspring sired by a zebra whose later offspring were striped). This idea contradicted August Weismann's influential hypothesis that the germline (determined by genetic inheritance) could not be influenced by individual physiology (soma). The Weismann principle of a barrier ensuring continuity of the germline, formulated in 1872 and long considered a basic tenet of biology, asserted the absolute independence of DNA from environmental influences (generally known as the Mendelian inheritance model) and the impossibility of individual adaptations acquired over a lifetime becoming hereditary traits (the phenomenon known as Lamarckism).

McLaren had her doubts and set to work mid-century on a series of elegant experiments designed to test the maternal transmission theory. She had to start largely from scratch, and the work was intensely laborious. Peering into her micro-scope day and night examining tiny fertilised mouse eggs in her University College lab, surrounded by home-made shoebox mouse houses and piles of battered lab books, few would have guessed the 25 year old would successfully challenge two of the most influential dogmas of twentieth-century genetics: the separation of ger-mline and soma, and its later molecular corollary – the one-way coding of DNA. Nor could anyone have predicted, even if they knew the goal of her research, that McLaren, along with her colleague John Biggers, were also quietly perfecting one of the most important experimental technologies of the twentieth century – namely mammalian embryo transfer. It is therefore worth pausing briefly to return to this unusual experimental trajectory, which also helped to usher in successful human IVF, because it not only helps us to understand McLaren's contribution to the Warnock Committee three decades later, but also how 'human fertilisation and embryology' became one of the most important but underestimated translational landscapes of the past half-century.

Translating Embryo Transfer

Embryo transfer has many histories, including in plants, marine organisms and birds but it is particularly challenging in mammals, whose reproductive systems are comparatively inaccessible both physically and visually. Beginning as a re-search technique in experimental embryology in the nineteenth century, embryo transfer was only rarely used in mammals until the mid-twentieth century (Franklin 2013). McLaren was an exception to this pattern, along with several others, and between 1952 and 1958 she and her husband Donald Michie – having recently completed their doctorates in Zoology at Oxford – gradually succeeded in refining mammalian embryo transfer to investigate the elusive biological mechanisms link-ing uterine gestation to genetic inheritance. What might the transfer of a 'donor' fertilised egg from one mouse to another reveal about the physiological interaction between a foster mother and her offspring – or a re-implanted embryo and its new parent? What could be learned about the intricate relationship between gestation and genetics during the most formative early stages of mammalian development by criss-crossing embryos in this way? Would it even be possible to use this technique on a sufficient scale to answer such fundamental questions? And what else might it reveal?

Over the seven years McLaren studiously performed her meticulous series of disruptive experiments using tiny hand-made surgical tools, and diligently record-ing the results of hundreds of cycles of transfers in her lab books, it would not have been at all apparent – even to her – what a momentous union between reproduc-tion, technology and scientific understanding was unfolding beneath her patient gaze. Belied by the simplicity of the concept of comparing the fates of native and transferred mouse embryos were technical and theoretical challenges so demand-ing they remain at the core of biomedical research today – half a century later in a world that has seen reproductive biology become one of the largest and most suc-cessful subfields of the life sciences.

Like many era-redefining experiments, the highly technical language of McLaren and Michie's scientific papers on embryo transfer, published between 1954 and 1961, gives little away. References to 'artificial' ovulation induction and to 'transmigration' of embryos, as well as to 'reciprocal crosses' and 'donor eggs', however, hint at the enduring questions about biological development and inheritance, as well as reproduction and animal health, that continue to concern livestock breeders, scientists, clinicians, governments, entrepreneurs and policy makers today. Donald Michie's training as a statistician, and his use of complex mathematical formulas to reveal biological patterns, perfected during his work as a codebreaker alongside Alan Turing at Bletchley Park during the war, anticipated both the future of artificial machine intelligence modelled on living systems (such as embryos) and the use of biocomputing to map DNA. McLaren's ingenious embryo transfer experimentation paved the way not only for *in vitro* fertilisation (IVF), intracytoplasmic spermatic injection (ICSI), cloning by somatic cell nuclear transfer, human admixed embryos and preimplantation genetic testing (PGT), but also human embryonic stem cell research and the new fields of *in vitro* gametogenesis (making sperm and eggs from stem cells) and embryo modelling. Her technical genius was never purely instrumental: the mastery of technique and ability to invent new tools and methods that characterised her lifelong effort to unravel the very earliest stages of mammalian development was driven by a visionary and unorthodox approach to biological complexity.

The iconoclastic style of research shared by McLaren and Michie – through which bold questions were pursued using unorthodox methods and techniques – not only shaped their science: it also reflected their political and social outlook, as well as their desire for science to serve as a progressive source of social change and solidarity. Like many of their generation who witnessed the radical overturning of so many established conventions and social norms in the aftermath of two world wars, they were free to imagine brave new possibilities for improving human futures. As paid-up members of the Communist Party, campaigners against nuclear weapons and trade union activists, McLaren and Michie's political views were orientated towards radical change. The benefits of scientific and technological progress, as well as international collaboration to deliver them, and public trust in their value as a social good, played key roles in their vision of a better, healthier, freer, wiser and more harmonious society, to which they were both keen to contribute.

Mixed Breeding

McLaren's long series of embryo transfer experiments between 1952 and 1958 embodied all of these goals. The technique itself criss-crossed between scientific, medical and agricultural applications, and addressed complex theoretical as well as practical problems. Embryo transfer was at once a classical and an obscure technique, first performed in mammals by the Mancunian polymath and embryologist Walter Heape in 1890. The son of a wealthy textile merchant, Heape took his early scientific training at Owens College, an early Polytechnique that later became the University of Manchester. Here, in one of the most prosperous cities in England,

Heape's formal education emphasised the rich mix of science, innovation and commerce that had fuelled the region's meteoric rise during the industrial revolution. His own chosen path of scientific research reflected this union of utility, inventiveness and economy in a series of embryo transfer experiments that, like McLaren's, were both ingenious and practical, with commercial as well as conceptual implications. The experiments Heape designed had to overcome daunting technical challenges, requiring skills and expertise drawn from animal husbandry, zoology and medicine as well as embryology, anatomy and physiology. As a Cambridge research scientist, and later as a Fellow of the Royal Society, Heape's goal was to contribute to basic biological science. But he was equally a product of his pragmatic Mancunian upbringing, with an eye on industry and commerce as well as scholarly publication.

Embryo transfer was to the late nineteenth century what embryo models are to twenty-first-century scientists seeking to understand the elaborate interaction between heredity, development and reproduction: it was a hugely helpful investigative technique. It was particularly useful for a whole host of unanswered scientific and practical questions about the precise mechanisms linking one generation to the next. Livestock breeders were understandably keen to ensure that desired traits be passed on and preserved, so that valuable animals could be reliably bred to maximise their most highly prized qualities. Better scientific knowledge of maternal and paternal roles in reproduction, as well as the mechanisms of hereditary transmission, would greatly aid this task by revealing the basic biological principles that could ensure greater control of hereditary transmission. But Heape's successful experiments also shed light on fundamental questions about the development of the germline that were of fundamental importance to basic science.

From its inception, then, embryo transfer occupied a pivotal place between both theory and practice, and reproduction and heredity. Three years after Heape published his embryo transfer experiments in the *Proceedings of the Royal Society* in 1906, the Danish pharmacist and plant biologist Wilhelm Johannsen would coin the words 'gene', 'genotype' and 'phenotype' to replace the concept of 'pangene' introduced by Darwin to describe the 'elements' or 'hereditary particles' through which intergenerational traits were passed on. One year later, following in Heape's footsteps, the Cambridge biologist Francis Hugh Adam Marshall published the first edition of the field-defining textbook *The Physiology of Reproduction* in 1910. Here, for the first time, and in compendious detail, the attempt to map the complex interactions between gametes, genes, gestation, hormones, nutrition, parturition and heredity was undertaken on an unprecedented scale. The book is still in print, having expanded from one to four volumes, and remains both a foundational text and a testament to the breadth and influence of the field it spawned.

Throughout the first half of the twentieth century, the 'disciplining' of reproduction proceeded apace. As the feminist historian Adele Clarke illustrates in her landmark volume documenting the influential social and scientific worlds of reproductive control that emerged during the half-century following the publication of Marshall's text, this was a period in which saw 'profound changes in the orientations not only of reproductive scientists but also of their key sponsors and markets'

(Clarke 1998: 6). By 'disciplining', Clarke refers both to the emergence of a new scientific field – reproductive biology – but also to the way in which the biology of reproduction could be more effectively controlled using new scientific techniques. From the hybridisation of corn and other industrialised plant breeding methods to the introduction of artificial reproduction into livestock programmes – and the successful design of new birth control methods for human use – increased biological control based on the application of scientific principles to the reproductive systems of humans, animals, plants and microorganisms is a major theme of the new world order that emerged in the twentieth century.

The 1960s were a period during which many of these trajectories both converged and intensified: anxiety about population growth fuelled new agricultural initiatives such as the Green Revolution, while techniques used for livestock breeding migrated ever more rapidly into applications to control human fertility. The concept of 'artificial' reproduction expanded from experiments designed to replicate and model natural processes to more instrumental means of manipulating reproductive outcomes for industrial as well as medical purposes. Positioned as they were, on the cusp of a new era in which techniques developed by experimental embryologists in the nineteenth century would be reborn as the technological platforms enabling an unprecedented industrialisation of fertility, scientists working in the fields of reproductive and developmental biology were right to expect that major changes were in store for humans as well as rabbits, mice and sheep. As population control rose on the agenda of global planning organisations such as the World Bank and the International Monetary Fund, major research foundations such as Rockefeller, Ford and Carnegie increasingly directed huge sums into reproductive research and embryology.

Experimental Transfers

Just over a century after his birth in 1855, Heape's embryo transfer legacy is celebrated in the opening paragraph of Anne McLaren and Donald Michie's 1956 article, published in the prestigious *Journal of Experimental Biology*, outlining all the ways this pivotal technique might be expanded to address a wide range of problems 'in genetics, embryology, reproductive physiology, immunology and cancer research [as well as] livestock farming'. Opening their article with a detailed description of Heape's experimental transfer of two fertilised eggs from an Angora doe rabbit to a Belgian hare rabbit, leading to the birth of two offspring resembling their donor Angora mother, and four resembling the Belgian surrogate host, they note the unique value of this technique as both a scientific tool and an agricultural application – while also gesturing toward its potential value to medical science and clinical care.

A century on from their Victorian precursor in Manchester, McLaren and Michie had the advantages of more advanced scientific knowledge, better equipment, and new techniques of cell culture to help handle the tiny microscopic mouse egg cells they needed to collect, preserve, manipulate and document in large numbers for their experiments. But embryo transfer in mice was not for the fainthearted. Over and over, using tiny pipettes, McLaren would collect, count, record and then corral her precious batch of fertilised mouse eggs in the centre of a watch-glass filled with Ringer-phosphate saline, readying them for pick-up and transfer into the oviducts of recipient, hormonally synchronised surrogates – a complex series of delicate operations laced with hazards. This demanding micro technical routine had to be exactly repeated hundreds of times in tight coordination with the reproductive cycles of the donor and recipient mice. As in the past, embryo transfer potentially offered a crucial means of disaggregating various factors affecting the development of fertilised eggs, such as how many eggs were transferred at one time, which oviduct (left or right) they were transferred into, whether 'alien' and 'native' eggs were present in the same or different oviducts, and at what stages of development the transfers took place. In turn, this knowledge helped to improve techniques such as ovulation induction and artificial insemination, while also shedding light on factors influencing both the success of embryo transfer and the very earliest stages of mammalian implantation. But it took considerable time, patience and persistence to make it work.

Throughout her distinguished scientific career, Anne McLaren would doggedly pursue the questions of how the egg develops, how to track its interactions with

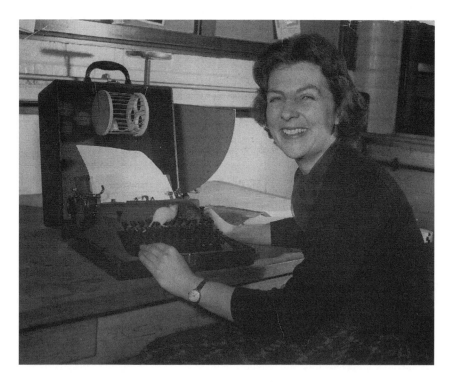

Figure 3.1 Dr Anne McLaren's lab research involved the use of embryo transfer in mice to pursue her lifelong research goal of 'understanding everything involved in getting from one generation to the next'.

its environment, and how these 'germinal' insights can be translated into improved reproductive outcomes for humans as well as other animals. Across a lifetime of scientific research that closely mirrored Heape's in its far-reaching and polymathic approach to reproductive science as a social mission, McLaren would contribute to a huge range of progressive social causes – from improving women's reproductive health and combatting genetic disease to building global scientific partnerships and creating ethical science policy. She was determined to deliver better understandings of 'everything involved in getting from one generation to the next'. Even as a biologist, her scientific interests were broad, eclectic and ambitious while at the same time her intellectual imagination stretched far beyond the life sciences to encompass concerns about society, ethics, policy and the law.

Key to both her vision of public science in the public interest and her zeal for communicating the vital role of scientific research in promoting social welfare was McLaren's belief that the benefits better science could generate were both obvious for non-scientists to appreciate, and self-evidently advantageous to society. The improvements to health, welfare, economy, efficiency, productivity, knowledge and understanding that successful scientific discovery and application could deliver were, in her view, crucial to not only human progress but to greater social equality, international collaboration, successful governance and welfare. Poverty, disease, war, famine and waste were just some of the major global challenges that not only could benefit from better scientific knowledge, but would absolutely require joined-up scientific and technological solutions on a global scale. They also required scientists to engage thoughtfully and meaningfully with a wide range of audiences, and to take seriously public concerns about new areas of scientific investigation, as well as the need for robust scientific governance and better science education. For both McLaren and Michie, as for their predecessor Heape, embryo transfer was not just about the transfer of embryos: it was about the transfer of improved scientific knowledge into practical applications, and thus the translation of better science into economic benefits, improved human health and progressive social change.

Mouse Lessons

Small as the minuscule mouse eggs she was studying may have been, there is no doubt Anne McLaren was focussed on big picture questions as she conducted her painstaking experiments in UCL between 1952 and 1955, and later at the Royal Veterinary College (RVC) in Camden, where she and Donald had to move in order to accommodate their ever-growing mousery. With another grant from the Agricultural Research Council, and now lodged in the former Fly Room (part of the Canine Block) at the RVC, Anne and Donald continued their epic five-year marathon to master embryo transfer and all its inter-related technical elements in order to finally determine what it could reveal about 'uterine' effects on offspring. This project had undoubted significance for basic science, embryological technique and agricultural applications. It also had obvious potential for human use and McLaren was already aware that her colleague Robert Edwards was also interested in this technique – in his case with a view to using it for human *in vitro* fertilisation. McLaren later explained in an interview that she 'realized that this technology we had in mice would probably eventually be applied to women too', and she went on to say:

> I was very keen that when *in vitro* fertilization or embryo transfer or whatever was successfully developed in women it should get a good press as it were and that women should realize that this was potentially beneficial for them and not be scared and suspicious of a new, strange technique and I suppose one realized eventually that it was more likely to be so when it was regulated.
>
> (McLaren 2004)

Tedious though the steady march through the embryo transfer experiments had proven to be, however, they were delivering results that would have tectonic conceptual as well practical reverberations. By the 1980s, McLaren would herself be working with NASA to send mouse embryos into outer space, and human *in vitro* fertilisation would be available on the NHS.

Despite its evident successes, however, the post-war birth of mammalian developmental biology was a lengthy parturition — complicated in part by the cellular changes revealed by the use of nuclear weapons which played a crucial role in the effort to transform wartime science into medical applications. 'Radiation Biology', as it came to be known, had already harnessed the power of X-rays to modify DNA and could be used as a valuable research tool to reveal otherwise indetectable biological mechanisms, promising to open up whole new research pathways – and in particular to help elucidate the precise mechanisms of genetic inheritance. As noted above, James Watson's research fellowship at Cambridge, where he pursued the structure of the double-helix alongside Francis Crick, was funded by the US Atomic Energy Commission, and Crick's lab, where the physical and chemical reproductive mechanisms of the double-helix were successfully modelled in 1953, was linked to the Cavendish Physics Laboratory, where James Clerk Maxwell had earlier discovered electro-magnetism and later Ernest Rutherford and his students parsed the elementary structures of atomic nuclei, magnetism, radioactivity, electricity and light. Although the impact on biology of DNA's structural unravelling would be slow, it would eventually transform the life sciences in the second half of the twentieth century, opening up a new era of molecular analysis of the foundational interactions between DNA, RNA and protein, and enabling completion of the first full map of the human genome by the century's end.

Much like embryo transfer, the molecular study of nuclear DNA's reproductive acrobatics in mammals is both laborious and unpredictable. It also requires complex experimental tools, methods, equipment and procedures – the development of which comprises a major part of the study of genomics. Like egg cells and embryos, DNA is not simply a carrier of information, or code, but a site of complex interactions. In contrast to the apparently obvious self-replicating mechanics of nuclear DNA's famous double helix, even simple aspects of the behaviour of its four chemical bases – such as which direction they coil while replicating, where they reside on the chromosome, and how they 'break', 'jump' and 'code' – remain under-characterised biological phenomena. Odd chromosomal fractures, duplications and 'transpositions' – when one part of the chromosome relocates in a manner that can become heritable – are of particular relevance to human medicine in terms of both health and reproduction. The often severe and potentially lethal developmental disorders caused by chromosomal trisomies and translocations, for example, as well as the debilitating and sometimes fatal inherited diseases caused by single gene mutations such as Tay Sachs or Thalassemia, are a major source of concern not only for parents and clinicians, but also for people who might be carriers thinking about having biological children. However, the much larger categories of congenital and chronic disease caused by environmental factors are not strictly non-genetic in origin – and indeed may, in some cases, be acquired by one generation who then transmit a hereditary tendency or trait to the next.

Brave New Mice

This is exactly the scenario Anne McLaren was studying in her London lab during the same period the structure of the double-helix was being investigated by her colleagues Rosalind Franklin and Maurice Wilkins down the road at King's College, and 50 miles away in Cambridge. As described at the outset of this chapter, her experiments were specifically designed to employ the embryo transfer technique to disaggregate genetic from environmental effects in mouse models. Since the immediate 'environment' of early mammalian embryos is the uterus – and the origins of germ cells and gametes are in the bodies of either one or both parents – biological interest has long been focussed on the question of how to track these developmental interactions more fully. Using two breeds of mice who differed in their number of sacral vertebrae, McLaren's hundreds of experimental embryo transfer cycles combined with Donald Michie's high-level statistical analysis finally revealed definitive proof of their hypothesis that the mother's body could, in fact, 'reprogramme' DNA. Following a period of elegant and meticulous experimentation lasting more than five years, the results were published in *Nature* in 1958 under the title 'An Effect of the Uterine Environment upon Skeletal Morphology in the Mouse' (McLaren and Michie 1958).

A photograph of Anne taken in the same year shows her seated in front of her manual typewriter in her laboratory in the Canine Block, with a small white mouse cavorting on an exercise wheel inside its lid. Now herself a parent, with a toddler and an infant often accompanying her to the lab, Anne was busy expanding her embryo transfer work in multiple directions. Following her move in 1955 to larger quarters, she was motivated by the success of a new culture media system in the lab of an adjacent scientist, John Biggers, and together they began a series of experiments to investigate additional aspects of maternal influence. Their aim was to shed light on the effects of environment on the embryos of different strains of mice and to do so Biggers cultured the fertilised mouse eggs to blastocyst stage before transferring them to surrogates. The success of this methodology – the production of 'bottled' baby mice – immediately captured media attention. Anne and John's

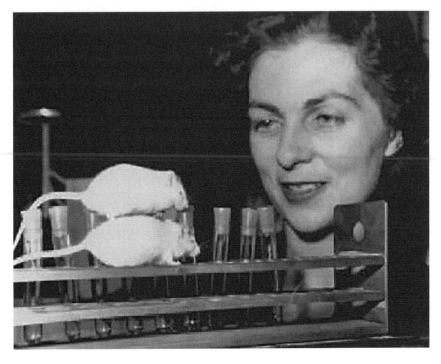

Figure 3.2 McLaren's early work with Professor John Biggers at University College London paved the way for clinical human IVF – a technique she foresaw as bringing significant benefits to women and couples suffering from involuntary childlessness.

Letter to *Nature* in November of 1958 entitled 'Successful birth and development of mice cultivated *in vitro* as early embryos' prompted an article in *The Telegraph* entitled 'Brave New Mice'.

'Test-tube babies', the article claims, have come even closer with the help of UCL scientists who are successfully culturing embryos in glass before transferring them to surrogate mothers. 'If methods continue to improve', the *Telegraph* science correspondent Anthony Smith surmised, it would be possible to conduct beneficial scientific research on embryos that would previously have been impossible. True to his prediction, the long-awaited test-tube baby was indeed imminent. Within a year, Min Chueh Chang from the Worcester Foundation for Experimental Biology in central Massachusetts would confirm in a letter to *Nature* the first successful fertilisation of a rabbit egg *in vitro*.

It would be yet another decade before Robert Edwards, having managed to combine in humans many of the exact same procedures McLaren, Michie and Biggers had earlier perfected in mice at UCL, and Chang had first proved possible in Worcester, would publish a letter in *Nature*, co-authored with his PhD student Barry Bavister and his medical collaborator Patrick Steptoe (Edwards et al. 1969), announcing the 'early stages of fertilisation *in vitro* of human oocytes matured *in vitro*', and concluding that there 'may be certain clinical and scientific uses for human eggs fertilized by this procedure'. Nearly another decade would pass until July 1978, when Louise Brown became the first 'test-tube baby' to be born, at Kershaw Hospital in Oldham, Lancashire, where Edwards and Steptoe, along with their project coordinator Jean Purdy and a vast team of nursing and technical support, had finally managed to transfer IVF and embryo transfer into human clinical use.

Conclusion

From her earliest experiments in mice, Anne McLaren was not only concerned with answering basic scientific questions about reproduction and heredity, inventing new methods to do so, and translating these into new applications. She was also keen to promote the social benefits of good science and to ensure the public could understand, appreciate and value them. As her prescient understanding of IVF and embryo transfer demonstrate, she also understood that the general public would be less likely to be 'scared and suspicious' of a 'new and strange technique' if it was positively depicted in the media and well regulated.

Unlike molecular genetics, the science of artificial reproduction that began to accelerate in the mid-twentieth century quickly acquired huge translational significance. The introduction of the oral contraceptive pill was only the first of many successful translational reproductive technologies. Livestock breeding was transformed at an industrial level – and globally – by the new techniques of artificial insemination, cryopreservation, IVF and embryo transfer. These highly successful agricultural technologies opened the door not only for similar clinical applications in humans but established the IVF platform as a fundamental research tool in the life sciences. Cloning, stem cell technologies and more recently embryo modelling are all the offspring of the migration of IVF from basic science into agriculture and from there into the clinic.

As Anne McLaren also clearly understood, successful scientific translation is not simply a matter of building a better mouse model. To succeed, new technologies need not only to be accepted – but trusted, valued and appreciated (Franklin 2007). Both 'disciplining' and translating reproduction are ultimately social and political projects, as well as scientific ones. As her work also shows, IVF is not only a bridge between *in vivo* and *in vitro* biology, or a link to understanding the intimate choreography linking gametogenesis to inheritance, and vice versa. It is also a bridge between basic science, better health and new applications such as *in vitro*-derived gametes, mitochondrial donation, regenerative medicine and pre-implantation genetic testing. Further than this, IVF has also turned out to be a crucial bridge between science and its many publics – indeed so much so that it is today a unique signifier of this connection. This is perhaps the most important reason of all why thinking through the lens of IVF is not only significant biologically, medically and scientifically – but also sociologically, ethically and in terms of governance and policy.

As we shall see in later chapters, these are lessons both Anne McLaren and Mary Warnock not only understood but put into action on behalf of good science, and science as a social good, as well as communication and outreach about science. The Warnock social contract that underlies the UK's human fertilisation and embryology legislation both expresses and embodies this view. Consequently it is helpful to be reminded of yet another important lesson from the history of IVF which is how intimately all of these different kinds of thinking, reasoning and communicating are interconnected in the process of successful translation.

References

Chang, Min Chueh (1959) 'Fertilization of rabbit ova *in vitro*' *Nature* 184(4684): 466–467.

Clarke, Adele E. (1998) *Disciplining reproduction: modernity, American life sciences, and the problems of sex* (University of California Press).

Edwards, R.G., Bavister, B.D. and Steptoe, P.C. (1969) 'Early stages of fertilization *in vitro* in human oocytes matured *in vitro*' *Nature* 221(5181): 632–635.

Franklin, Sarah (2007) 'Obituary: Dame Dr Anne McLaren' *Regenerative Medicine* 2(5): 853–859.

Franklin, Sarah (2013) *Biological relatives: IVF, stem cells and the future of kinship* (Duke University Press).

Hart, Julian Tudor (2010) *The political economy of health care: where the NHS came from and where it could lead* (Policy Press).

Heape, Walter (1897) 'The artificial insemination of mammals and subsequent possible fertilization or impregnation of their ova' *Proceedings of the Royal Society London* 61(369–377): 52–63.

Johannsen, W. (1909) *Elemente der exakten Erblichkeitslehre* [*Elements of the exact theory of heredity*] (Gustav Fischer).

Keller, Evelyn Fox (2003) *Making sense of life: explaining biological development with models, metaphors and machines* (Harvard University Press).

Marshall, Francis Hugh Adam, Cramer, William and Lochhead, James (1910) *The physiology of reproduction* (Longmans, Green and Company).

McLaren, Anne (2004) 'A conversation with Dr Anne McLaren, DBE, DPhil, FRS, FRCOG' *Human Fertility* 7(2): 83–89.

McLaren, Anne, and Biggers, J.D. (1958) 'Successful development and birth of mice cultivated *in vitro* as early embryos' *Nature* 182(4639): 877–878.

McLaren, Anne and Michie, Donald (1956) 'Studies on the transfer of fertilized mouse eggs to uterine foster-mothers, I: factors affecting the implantation and survival of native and transferred eggs' *Journal of Experimental Biology* 33(2): 394–416.

McLaren, Anne, and Michie, Donald (1958) 'An effect of the uterine environment upon skeletal morphology in the mouse' *Nature* 181(4616): 1147–1148.

McLaren, Anne, and Michie, Donald (1959) 'Studies on the transfer of fertilized mouse eggs to uterine foster-mothers, II: the effect of transferring large numbers of eggs' *Journal of Experimental Biology* 36(1): 40–50.

4   The Legislative Origins of the 14 Day Rule

No one had ever legislated in the novel area of 'human fertilisation and embryology' when Mary Warnock was appointed in 1982 to chair a committee responding to the birth of the world's first test-tube baby in 1978. To complicate matters, IVF was not the only technique included in the Warnock Committee's expansive brief 'to examine the social, ethical and legal implications of recent and potential developments in the field of human assisted reproduction'. Other areas requiring regulation included surrogacy, egg and sperm donation and storage, artificial insemination, and the national regulation of infertility services as well as embryo research (Warnock 1985). Because these were matters of 'special' moral significance, and considerable legal uncertainty, the Committee would have to consider ethical philosophical questions alongside legal, regulatory and scientific matters in order to devise a viable political strategy through which to implement successful regulation. This would require 'filling a legal vacuum' as no legislation of 'human fertilisation and embryology' had ever been devised before.

This challenge was exacerbated by the shifting political climate, in which issues related to social morality, such as abortion, homosexuality and censorship were once more at the forefront of public and media attention. The election of Margaret Thatcher in 1979 and Ronald Reagan a year later in the United States helped to fuel a resurgence of moral conservatism, and in the UK a 'return to traditional family values' was widely celebrated by opponents of the progressive changes introduced in the 1960s and 70s, and the loosening of restrictions on homosexuality, divorce, contraception and abortion. Predictably, and from the outset, the regulation of assisted conception was seized upon by conservative pressure groups as an opportunity to overturn the 1967 Abortion Act. Parliamentary calls for a Committee of Inquiry to investigate the social, legal and medical implications of *in vitro* fertilisation ominously invoked its potential to 'imperil the dignity of the human race, threaten the welfare of children, and destroy the sanctity of family life' (Lord Campbell, HL Deb 9 July 1982). It was consequently evident well in advance of the final confirmation of its membership, chair and terms of reference that one of the main difficulties the Warnock Committee would immediately encounter – if not its primary obstacle – would be avoiding the highly polarised abortion debate.

At the time the members of the Warnock Committee began their negotiations in the autumn of 1982, it was unclear whether a majority of the public, or of Parliament,

DOI: 10.4324/9781003294108-4

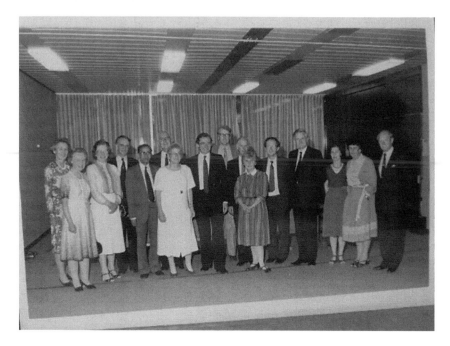

Figure 4.1 The Warnock Committee: the 16 Members of the Inquiry were supported by two
key administrators as well as a large staff of civil servants.

supported embryo research or IVF.[1] While a vocal minority of hard-line religious
activists strongly opposed IVF and embryo research, it was much harder to determine how the general public viewed such novel scientific innovations. On the
Committee itself, unanimous support for most techniques, including IVF, was not
matched with equal willingness to allow research on embryos – particularly those
created for research purposes – and ultimately 7 of the 16 members would dissent
on this matter, which proved to be the most controversial single issue the Warnock
Committee had to wrestle with throughout its two year deliberations.

The means by which the Committee members debated the science of embryology thus became a central focus for both Warnock and McLaren. Careful examina-
tion of the strategies Warnock and McLaren employed to reach the desired goal of
maximally permissive but unusually strict legislation reveals a sensitivity to social
and cultural factors that anticipates many of today's challenges in the context of
translational technologies involving embryos. Because embryo research became
the somewhat unexpected flashpoint for basic questions about morality, ethics,
religion, politics, law and science, the option of a purely scientific basis for the
Committee's deliberations was precluded from the outset. At the same time, precise and well-established scientific definitions of embryological development were
essential not only in order for the Committee's decisions to be regarded as rigorous,
credible and authoritative, but specifically so that a clear bright line could be drawn
on which viable regulation could be based. Above all what was needed was factual

groundwork on which to build a popular and parliamentary consensus large and strong enough to prevail against a well-organised campaign of religious opposition to embryo research and IVF that had deep roots in both Parliament and the Conservative Party. Repeatedly, the idiom of 'drawing a line' was used to describe both a pragmatic requirement for general clarity, and a strategy for delivering a sustainable progressive policy toward research into human fertilisation and embryology.

Biological Translation

As we shall see, however, the question of 'where to draw the line' paradoxically refers both to the arbitrariness of boundaries, and the necessity for a division between one thing and another to be both absolute and obvious. While a 'line' can refer to a limit or cut-off point, it can also refer to what McLaren preferred to call 'landmarks' – meaning established and well-characterised biological transition points in early human development. A 'landmark' is conventionally defined as a signpost marking a path, a border, or a well-known material object by means of which it is possible to determine one's location. Figuratively, a 'landmark' can describe a turning point, or transition, as in the case of a 'landmark discovery' such as penicillin. For Warnock, these two definitions needed to be merged: she needed literal scientific landmarks to establish a path to guide her Committee toward a hypothetical regulatory framework that could be based on precise scientific facts, but also enacted as a general set of laws. Likewise, McLaren was convinced that 'developmental 'landmarks' were essential in order to establish an authoritative scientific and factual foundation for the moral reasoning on which firm legal guidelines – and a clear bright line – could be based. But marshalling all of these logics together into seamless alignment was never going to be straightforward.

However, if the means were not obvious, the objective was crystal clear: within less than 24 months, the Committee would need to deliver a comprehensive, persuasive, policy-friendly and clearly signposted roadmap to Parliament for the future regulation and governance of 'human fertilisation and embryology' in the wake of successful human IVF. This meant they had to be relentlessly focussed on achieving a viable consensus around a workable regulatory strategy, which would be as encompassing and future-proof as possible. Always for Warnock, the far-sighted Committee Chair, a primary concern was to avoid being lured down either the rabbit-hole of 'the moral status of the human embryo' or the *cul de sac* of the highly polarised abortion debate, and instead to guide her members toward the less divisive moral terrain of deliberative justice, where a viable compromise could be carefully composed on the basis of reasoned argument rather than religious doctrine. According to Warnock's pragmatic moral compass, a complete ban on IVF and embryo research would be indefensible and reactionary – and was therefore an outcome that should be avoided as fervently as the possibility of an unbreachable impasse that would lead to no legislation at all.

Equally vital from the outset of the Committee's deliberations was Warnock's clear-sighted forecast that in order for either IVF or embryo research to be allowed, there would need to be firm limits and prohibitions that were both persuasive and rigorous. Compromises would be essential because fundamental disagreements would be unavoidable, but the end result had to be a regulatory system that inspired the highest confidence among the widest audience. This was what we would now describe as an explicitly 'translational' goal. Supporting scientific progress in aid of improved reproductive medicine, Warnock believed, was morally right, but would require cast-iron ethical and legal governance in order to become socially and politically – as well as legally – acceptable, governable and thus clinically viable. With the benefit of much committee work behind her, Warnock prioritised reasoned consensus as her goal, and set about designing a regulatory framework based on an exchange: in exchange for allowing research into human fertilisation and embryology to continue, and for further clinical and scientific benefits to be explored, the very highest levels of regulatory vigilance, control and sanctions had to be both present and enforceable. Clear legislative restrictions to scientific research would enable its benefits to be maximised while its risks and future direction could be transparently governed. Such an achievement would not only deliver the best outcome for the most people, including future generations, but would set an example of best practice in terms of non-partisan regulatory practice.

To deliver a means of regulating potentially beneficial but controversial scientific practice in this way would not only have many practical benefits. As noted earlier, it would also, Warnock believed, express 'a moral idea of society' in the form of establishing 'some barriers that are not to be crossed' and thus 'the minimum requirement for a tolerable society' (Warnock Committee 1984: paras 5–6). This was an ambitious bio-translational goal: in order for potentially controversial bioscientific discoveries to become not only successful clinical applications, but publicly trusted and valued contributions to health, medicine and society, they typically have to undergo a lengthy period of being 'bedded in' – both literally at patients' bedsides and in the more general sense of being normalised as accepted, legitimate and trustworthy treatments. As Warnock rightly judged from the outset, public acceptance of new reproductive technologies like IVF, and controversial areas of scientific research such as human embryo experimentation, would depend not only on what people knew about these technologies but also what they *felt* about them. The same was true for her Committee members: they would need not only to be taught how to make sense of the complex stages of embryonic development, and to incorporate these understandings into some kind of regulatory framework, but be enabled to feel confident with the lines of reasoning used to justify their recommendations, as well as the lines demarcating the permissible from the impermissible in the brave new world of 'bottled babies'.

In sum, Mary Warnock needed her fellow Committee members to find as much common ground as possible upon which to base a new social contract for reproductive biomedicine. Moreover, in order to fill the 'legal vacuum' that existed in the wake of Louise Brown's birth, Warnock needed a convincing outline of clear legal principles, guidelines and procedures as well as a pragmatic account of how regulatory bodies would enforce them. Her Committee's recommendations would require high levels of parliamentary and professional as well as public approval, so they had to be built on a firm, confident, coherent and transparent set of reasonings.

To succeed in such a goal would 'fully translate' technologies such as IVF and embryo transfer not only into regular public use, but into the public consciousness as valued innovations – whose benefits outweighed their risks, and whose regulation they could trust. To secure this ambitious bio-translational goal would be even more complex than embryo transfer, requiring not only a wide range of professional skills, and diverse forms of expertise, but an astute ability to read the room, plan ahead and steer the boat to shore.

Around the Table

On 9 November 1983, all but one of the 16 Members of the Committee of Inquiry into Human Fertilisation and Embryology attended their twelfth monthly meeting in Hannibal House, the iconic London headquarters of the former Department of Health and Social Services (DHSS) based in Elephant and Castle. A single issue was the subject of the entire day's discussion, namely whether to permit any experimentation on human embryos, and if so under what conditions.

A briefing note to Mary Warnock, from the Committee Secretary, Jenny Croft, summarised the 'Organisation of the Day's Business' and anticipated some of the possible outcomes of this pivotal meeting: 'As agreed at the last meeting [13 October 1983], the whole of Wednesday is to be devoted to a discussion of experiments on embryos … We had thought in terms of allowing the morning for the more general discussion, and turning to the matters requiring decisions after lunch.'

She continued:

It may be that we cannot get answers to all the questions at the meeting, but I think we agreed we might need more than one meeting on the subject [as] it is a topic where it is important that the inquiry feel satisfied with the position they eventually take. If it would be helpful, we could draw together the lines of discussion on Wednesday, and any decisions which are reached into a connected piece of narrative for the next meeting [in December], so that members could consider whether this indeed represents their views.

Several briefing papers were prepared by the Committee Secretariat for the 9 November meeting. To open the discussion, a single-page document entitled 'Correspondence Analysis' (Paper 64) summarised the correspondence received by the Committee to date. A neat numeric table containing a sobering set of sum totals greeted the 16 members of the Inquiry assembled around the table in Hannibal House. Against only 8 letters written in support of IVF, 123 letters had been received by the Inquiry opposing either IVF or surrogacy, while yet another 284 letters specifically objected to experiments on embryos. In total, fifty times as many letters had been submitted in opposition to IVF, surrogacy and embryo experiments than those in favour.[2]

This was an unpromising set of figures with which to begin a meeting intended to establish a more permissive climate for IVF and embryo research. Indeed, observing these totals, few would have anticipated that within a decade the UK would

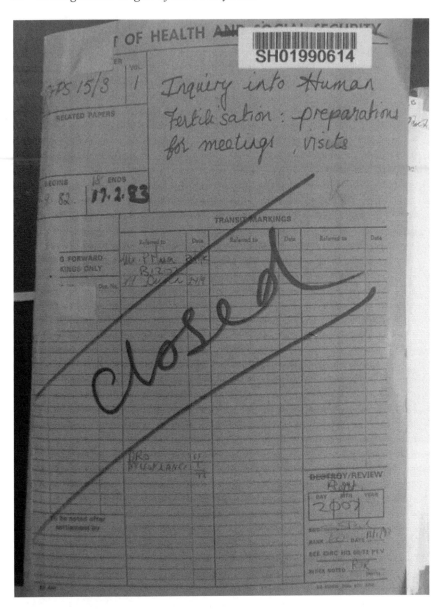

Figure 4.2 The original Warnock Committee files, which were embargoed for 30 years, from 1984 to 2014, and remain incomplete, were discovered in the Department of Health Repository in Burnley, Lancashire, in January 2016 by members of Cambridge's Reproductive Sociology Research Group (ReproSoc).

become home to one of the most supportive climates for reproductive biomedicine, where IVF was a household word. As a starting point for discussing their most challenging issue, on which, as Warnock later wrote, 'there is bound to be criticism that we have gone too far, or not far enough' (1985: vii), such a large 'no vote' from the public must have felt like a shot across the bows. Since only a small minority of Committee members favoured a ban on IVF and embryo research, the placement of this document at the top of the agenda signalled a call to arms. 'Time to get serious', Warnock appeared to be urging her Committee.

Two other papers, 'Therapy and Research' (Paper 58) and 'Other Areas Where Research Is Controlled' (Paper 61) contained factual background information prepared by the Secretariat for the November meeting. 'Therapy and Research' clarifies the distinctions between embryos created for different kinds of research, in order to help determine whether restrictions on embryo research should be the same for all of them. Paper 57, 'Experiments on Embryos: Key Questions', summarises the Inquiry's discussion of embryo research so far, reconfirming some of the key terms that have already been agreed, and matters that are no longer up for debate. For example, the Committee has already agreed, Paper 57 reminds them, on a working definition of 'embryo': 'for the practical purposes of the Inquiry the embryonic stage of development [will] be taken to cover the period from fertilisation until the end of the 8th week of gestation'. Similarly, in section 3 concerning 'the central issue', members are reminded that 'the question is not, as members have said on a number of occasions, when does life begin, which the Inquiry has agreed is a matter of belief as much as science'. The question instead is 'what moral status should be afforded an embryo, and hence what degree of protection, if any, should it be given'. As we see later, the question of moral status was also fraught with difficulty, leading the Committee to focus instead on the latter question, of what can legitimately be done to the human embryo.

'Views from the Evidence' goes on to contrast 'two main strands of opinion' concerning experiments on embryos, namely one that opposes them entirely, and another which is 'essentially utilitarian and pragmatic' and in favour of the benefits such research could bring. Among the proponents of the latter position, the paper continues, it is recognised that 'if such research is to be accepted by the general public, it must be performed within certain clearly defined limits and subject to external scrutiny', adding that:

> Although supporters of this approach often suggest a cut-off point after which no experiments should be permitted, these points tend to derive from practicalities such as the length of time an embryo can, in the present state of knowledge, be sustained *in vitro*, rather than on any view as to a qualitative difference in the embryo before and after the chosen point.
>
> (Paper 57: 2–3)

Emphasising the 'somewhat arbitrary nature of these cut-off points, since the rationale for their existence could be overturned by a breakthrough in technology', Paper 57 adds that a similarly unlikely basis for easy line-drawing is the difference between 'pure' and 'therapeutic' research, as outlined in Paper 58.

> Relatively few of those submitting evidence accepted the need for 'pure' research designed only to enhance knowledge. However, in many ways the distinction between therapy and pure research is spurious, since it is often

essential to advance the level of knowledge before it is possible to devise an experiment which has a direct therapeutic purpose. Thus, one cannot develop a gene probe until one knows how to detect the genetic material in a cell, and this has only proved possible through 'squashing' embryos in order to see what they are like. In practice, it is not possible to distinguish absolutely between pure and applied science.

(Paper 58: 2)

In the same way that a biological basis for limits can only be established by impos-ing arbitrary 'lines' or 'points' on what are essentially and obviously continuous processes of embryonic development, so too is the effort to distinguish between ba-sic research and clinical application a false premise since 'in practice' they too are part of a dynamic continuum. Indeed, they overlap so extensively there can never be any 'absolute' distinction between 'pure' and 'applied' research, and thus, by implication, some other way to 'draw a line' will be required in order to establish the limits on embryo research that will form the basis for policy.

Staging Development

In addition to Papers 57, 58, 62 and 64, two other papers were circulated with the minutes of the 9 November meeting. Paper 63, 'The funding of scientific re-search', outlines the role of the research councils and Paper 61 describes 'Other Areas Where Research is Controlled', including genetic manipulation, animal ex-periments, and dangerous pathogens. The final, and most important document, Pa-per 59, 'Research on Human Embryos *In vitro*, was also presented to the meeting.

Paper 59's summary of post-fertilisation embryonic development begins simply enough but quickly becomes more technical:

At fertilization the egg and sperm unite to become one toti potential cell with a single nucleus that contains the chromosomes derived from both parents. This single cell (or 'fertilized egg') then begins to divide rapidly into two, four, eight, sixteen cells, and so on. At this stage the cells hang together in a configuration similar to that of a blackberry. This is technically called a Morula.

Since it was unlikely that any Committee members would know the meaning of 'toti potential', its significance to development is clarified in subsequent para-graphs that explain the transition from morula to blastocyst stages, by which time 'the cells have lost their toti potential capacity', except for a portion called the in-ner cell mass, 'from which the embryo will be formed'. The rest of the blastocyst, 'although derived from the original fertilized egg and having the same genetic and chromosomal make-up', will not contribute cells 'to the embryo, fetus or child'.

The one-page 'simplified' summary of 'The Stages of Post Fertilisation De-velopment' accompanying the diagram in Annex A of Paper 59 is thus notable in its combined narration of the embryo *in toto* (from fertilised egg to morula to blastocyst) followed by its description and visual illustration of the emergence of

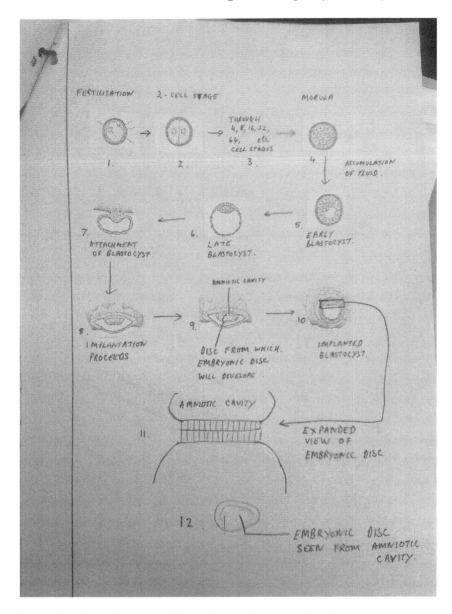

Figure 4.3 A linear illustration of the twelve earliest stages of embryonic development in humans is provided as Annex A of Paper 59, 'Research on Human Embryos *In Vitro*', prepared by the Secretariat for the 9 November 1983 meeting concerning 'where a line should be drawn' to limit research.

'the very small number of cells' that make up the inner cell mass, 'which continues to divide until an area within it can be identified as the "embryonic plate"'. The description concludes: 'Thus, it will be seen that the embryo (fetus and child) actually develop from a very small number of cells, all contained within the embryonic plate. The majority of cells of the pre-implantation embryo contribute to the formation of the placenta and fetal membranes but not to the embryo proper.' Crucial to this condensed account of post-fertilisation development is thus a division of the 'embryo' into two distinct entities: the 'pre-implantation embryo' (the whole embryo) and the 'embryo-proper' (the part of the inner cell mass that becomes the fetus and child).

This same division is clearly illustrated in the accompanying twelve-stage diagram that proceeds from fertilisation (1) through the two-cell stage (2); 4–64 cell stages (3); morula (4); early blastocyst (5); late blastocyst (6); attachment of blastocyst (to uterine wall, 7); implantation (8); and formation of the 'disc from which embryonic disc will develop' (9). Illustrations 10, 11, and 12 all depict the same stage – the formation of the embryonic disc – from different angles and in different scales.

The emphasis the diagram places on the embryonic disc is prominent and distinctive, and also conclusive, in that it concludes with an 'expanded view' of the division between the two sections of the developing embryo on about day eleven, which is drawn as a single line. Whereas the hand-drawn stages 1 through 8 are sequentially labelled and numbered, the depictions of stages 9 through 12 all illustrate one single stage in greater visual and textual detail: the formation of the embryonic disc. This self-evidently key stage is initially illustrated *in situ* within the implanted blastocyst (9–10), then at a larger scale (11), and finally from below (12). That the diagram culminates in an enlarged, multi-dimensional view of the embryonic disc's formation further underscores the sense of a key and clearly visible transition between one phase of development and another.

With the culminating emphasis of this Annex A diagram in mind, we can interpret the claim in Paper 59 that 'the majority of the cells in the pre-implantation embryo contribute to the formation of the placenta and fetal membranes but not to the embryo proper' even more pointedly, for it emerges that Papers 57 and 59 are concerned with not only key questions but also key divisions. Moreover, it is possible to read Annex A as a roadmap signposting the key developmental landmarks that could justify qualitative rather than practical cut-off points. In effect, and among other things, Paper 59 provides a neatly divided developmental narrative, which is reinforced both textually and diagrammatically in Annex A by an emphasis on key transitions. An overarching chronology of the biological development of a single embryo includes the morula, blastocyst, and post-implantation blastocyst stages familiar to the Committee since their first meeting, at which 'members agreed [that] the embryonic stage of development would be taken to cover the period from fertilisation until the end of the eighth week of gestation'. But a second, more specialised meaning of 'embryo' introduced in Papers 57 and 59 focuses on the subdivision of embryos themselves.

This second, more specialised definition becomes increasingly restrictive, including fewer and fewer cells as development progresses, marked by a series of divisions between different types of cells within the original fertilised egg. In the second paragraph of Annex A, 'embryo' initially means 'complete embryo', as in 'each toti potential cell might itself become a complete embryo'. This definition changes in paragraph 3: 'When the blastocyst forms it becomes clear which sections … include those cells from which the embryo will be formed'. This narrower definition is retained in paragraph 4, which explains that 'the rest of the blastocyst … will not contribute cells to the embryo, fetus or child'. The meaning of 'embryo' is narrowed still further in the final paragraph, in which the embryonic plate (or disc) becomes crucial because 'it is this part alone that contains the cells from which the embryo develops'. This point is immediately repeated: 'Thus it will be seen that the embryo (fetus and child) actually develop from a very small number of cells, all contained within the embryonic plate.' In a third iteration, the point is reinforced by introducing two new and important terms, the 'pre-implantation embryo' and the 'embryo proper': 'The majority of the cells in the pre-implantation embryo contribute to the formation of the placenta and fetal membranes, but not to the embryo proper.'

The 'Embryo Proper'

To understand the coming into being of the 'embryo proper' it is helpful to retrace its emergence across the key papers leading up to the crucial November meeting. They all emphasise, in both explicit and more subtle terms, the distinction introduced in the first paragraph of Paper 59 between 'research that might make use of human tissue which, though part of the embryonic sac, was not destined to become part of the embryo proper'. On page 3 of the same document, this distinction is again emphasised in reference to research on 'cells taken from those parts of the blastocyst that will not become part of the embryo proper'. The question of what kinds of research can be undertaken on which types of *in vitro*-fertilised embryos is thus recast as one of which parts of these same embryos have a different qualitative status. Therefore, qualitative criteria can take precedence over 'practicalities'.

After all, the issue for those attending the 9 November meeting was not the matter of research on embryos in general, but rather what kinds of research should be permitted on which types of embryos, and it is in a curious sentence in Paper 57 that this new ground for classifying embryos is initially named. The transformative, parenthetical sentence introduces a new distinction within the opening section of Paper 57 entitled 'The Meaning of "Embryo" in this Context':

(Strictly speaking fertilization results in a zygote which goes through morula and blastocyst stages, before the embryo proper can be identified as a discrete group of cells, but in considering the research issues this pre-embryonic period is very important as it is at this stage that *in vitro* development takes place).

This sentence not only introduces for the first time in the Warnock papers the concept of 'the embryo proper' to describe a 'discrete group of cells', but simultaneously inserts the equally transformative and crucial reference to a 'pre-embryonic period'. Intriguingly, this crucial sentence on the first page of a pivotal paper prepared for a critical meeting seems hastily written: the fifty-two-word insertion is poorly constructed, with a confusing reference to '*in vitro* development' (possibly a typographical error, since the likely intention was to refer to 'individual' development). The first sentence mentioning the 'embryo proper' thus appears to have been hurriedly inserted in order to revise a previously agreed upon definition of 'embryo' (as the first eight weeks of gestation) by first dividing early embryonic development into different stages (morula and blastocyst), and then replacing 'embryo' with the more specialised term 'zygote'. The turn to more technical language ('strictly speaking'), as well as the use of brackets, suggests the introduction of a *post facto* technical supplement to the broader definition of 'embryo' agreed upon at the Inquiry's outset (for 'practical purposes'). The second half of the sentence introduces an additional distinction between the embryo and 'the embryo proper', which is described as 'very important' in relation to the 'key questions' about embryo experimentation that will form the subject of the November meeting. The import of this new stage of embryonic development (should anyone remain in doubt) is accentuated by referencing a new timeline for the very earliest stages of human development, which now include the 'pre-embryonic period'.

The fact that Paper 57 was circulated in advance of 13 October 1983 meeting strongly suggests that an emergent form of biological reasoning based on the concept of 'the embryo proper' was already in use by the Secretariat prior to the November meeting. Paper 60, 'Defining the Limits for Research: Key Questions', was revised and distributed for the December meeting as Paper 64. 'At the November meeting of the Inquiry', it begins, 'members agreed to tackle the issues relating to research on human embryos in the following order: a) by type of embryo; b) by age of embryo; c) by category of research'. Like the earlier papers, 'Defining the Limits' offers a didactic summary, reminding the Committee members that at their previous meeting the most important 'developmental landmarks' had been identified, and that the result had been decisive: 'At the end of the meeting members had reached a view on whether research could be carried out on all but one type of embryo, those specially created for research purposes'.

Minutes from the December 1983 meeting similarly confirm that a clear set of landmarks were agreed at the November meeting as the basis for the Committee's recommendations, following almost exactly the path laid down in Annex A:

> Some members suggested a cut-off point of 14 days after fertilisation which they felt was widely regarded as a reasonable limit by the scientific community. At this date an *in vivo* embryo would have completed the implantation process. The 14-day embryo would have reached the point in development where the primitive streak had just begun to form at one end of the embryonic disk. Members decided that the limit for research should be 14 days. They decided that the formulation of the limit should be in the following terms: 'Not beyond the completion of the implantation stage or 14 days post fertilisation' and that it should also include a reference to the primitive streak.

Despite its odd, polyglot and anonymous composition, Annex A bears all the signs of being the product of a highly trained biologist with exactly McLaren's expertise – as well as the same principles she set out in the missing 'Where to Draw the Line' paper (and most likely introduced in the second meeting of the Authority in November 1982). Her ability to translate a specific developmental landmark – the point at which 'the primitive steak had begun to form at one end of the embryonic disc' – into the basis for viable and workable legislation was the result of both a cumulative and collective process. Warnock frequently praised McLaren's vital role on the Committee, crediting her superb communication skills, exemplified by her 'excellent diagrams' and 'non-intimidating manner which made the science available … to the wider public' as the secret of the Committee's success. She was equally effusive in her praise of Anne's 'genius as a teacher' and recalls with admiration her 'spellbinding powers of exposition and explanation', which she and many others relied upon extensively both during and after the Inquiry, as the Committee's recommendations passed gradually, but steadily and with minimal modification, into law. Clearly, McLaren was a skilled translator of biology, whose 'impeccable clarity', 'infinite patience' and 'unruffled amiability' enabled 'the developmental story of the fertilisation and post-fertilisation development of the embryo' to become the basis for the famous 14 day rule that has been described as the key translational pivot on which social consensus ultimately turned.

Interviewed in 2008 about the Committee's progress, Warnock described McLaren's translational role further in terms of providing a 'rationale' for 'a regulatory line' through which the 'crucial issue' for the Inquiry was 'solved':

[W]hat Anne had provided us with was a kind of rationale, I mean we could justify picking on that particular day, at fourteen days, because of what Anne had taught us about the development of the embryo and the date after conception at which differentiation began. And once we'd got that into our heads, then in a way, everything flowed from that … [O]nce you got a regulatory line beyond which, if you passed beyond which, you committed a criminal offence, then you needed some justification for having the line – the essential thing was to have a line. And so we didn't say anything like that the embryo before fourteen days or fifteen days, was completely different from the embryo after the fifteen days, we just told the story of the development of the embryo, the appearance of the primitive streak, the subsequent differentiation, and the fact, too, that identical twins could form up to fifteen days, all that – there's a sort of combined rationale for having put fourteen days as the time. But we desperately needed something, which you could count the days on the calendar and simply say, now this embryo's got to be destroyed. It was no good having a developmental point, because either some other scientist would come up and find another developmental point that was more important. Or somebody might say, well this is a, you know, is a late developing embryo or something. It would be disputable. Whereas, days one to fourteen could be marked off and you could just draw the line at that point. So once that crucial issue was solved, then we just stuck to the line and we knew that was what was going to go into the Report. And the only dissenters in that of course, were as I say, the people who on religious grounds, thought that the life of a human embryo was sacred from day nought really.

This passage is significant for several reasons, including Warnock's characteristically efficient summary of the three key facts about 'the story of the development of the embryo' that needed to be 'got ... into our heads' so that 'everything could flow from that'. These three 'developmental points' were 'the appearance of the primitive streak', 'the subsequent differentiation', and the fact that twins could form up until but not after this key dividing point in early human development. Crucially, however, these definitive transition points in and of themselves did not provide a sufficiently clear basis to 'just draw the line', according to Warnock, and her objective subtly shifts from finding 'a' rationale to developing a 'combined' rationale midway through, when the emphasis shifts to a 'regulatory line' and thus the need for a specific number: 'We desperately needed something [with] which you could count the days on the calendar', she explains. One line was not enough, it would appear – there had to be, in a sense, a numeric cut-off point to underline the biological one: 'It was no good having a developmental point' on its own because 'it would be disputable'. In contrast, 'one to fourteen could be marked off and you could just draw the line at that point'. In Warnock's view, 'once that crucial issue was solved, then we just stuck to the line and we knew that was what was going to go into the Report'.

The Committee secretary Jenny Croft similarly described the logical and practical challenges to setting a firm cut-off point in an interview about the Committee's debate over embryo research, describing them as 'tortuous':

You see, there isn't really a point at which the embryo becomes special. There really isn't. And therefore, justifying fourteen days is a bit tortuous, because you don't really want to say, we can't get them to last more than fourteen days, and that's what we're going for. Because then, when some clever person manages to keep them going for twenty-one, or whatever, you haven't got a justifiable position. So I think it's tortuous because it isn't really a justifiable position intellectually, you know, in the long run. ... I think most people on the Inquiry, and indeed, most of our correspondence insofar as that reflects the general public, were quite happy with the Louise Brown scenario. They thought that was exciting. It's once you started moving away from that, that people's feelings became fuzzy. And I think that part of the idea of the Inquiry was to put some definite parameters on that fuzziness. Unfortunately, it is by its nature, quite a fuzzy subject. And people's feelings change ... And so this whole thing was a rolling process, I think, of public awareness. And I suppose the success of the Inquiry was that it established a kind of [level] playing field, and it is still the research end that people are predominantly anxious about. I think they're still anxious for the reasons that we were anxious, because there [aren't any] clear lines. And people have an emotional feeling that human embryos ought to be special but [when] asked to define why, they can't, unless as I say, you go for the ultra-logical Catholic position of saying that they're, you know, that they're special from beginning to end. But a kind of English pragmatism suggests that that can't be right.

In her account of the 'fuzziness' surrounding the question of the 'point at which the embryo becomes special', Croft noticeably considers how people *feel* about the embryo as well as the logic behind various rationales for justifying a cut-off point. Her description of the 'tortuous' conflict between competing justifications not only emphasises the tension between an English pragmatism that favours support for scientific and technological progress and the 'ultra-logical' Catholic doctrine that life begins at conception. She also references the gap between a general public enthusiasm for IVF catalysed by the birth of Louise Brown and the anxiety shared by some Committee members and the public alike about embryo experimentation at a remove from the prospect of direct clinical benefits. Indeed she refers both repeatedly and specifically to the gap between 'emotional feeling' and an intellectual position regarding research on human embryos, which causes anxiety because of there are no 'clear lines'.

Croft also recalls the lingering tension between the need for a line to be drawn to enable the greater good of embryo research to become permissible and the acceptance by Committee members that no amount of logical evidence would ever definitively resolve 'whether that was right or not':

> Well, I think the committee accepted that a line had to be drawn at some point if they were going to allow any embryo research. And vaguely I can remember the occasion when the question of 'when is individuality established?' [came up]. It's when you don't, where you may end up with a disc with just one primitive streak, two primitive streaks or no primitive streak, but until that time you can't tell whether it's going to be one or nil or, unusually, two. I think Mary Warnock herself intervened at that time. So you can't actually tell whether there's individuality until that moment ... I think it was that argument that persuaded the bulk of the committee that fourteen days was as good a cut-off point as any. But they always recognised that there were going to be arguments as to whether that was right or not.

In this and many other descriptions of determining 'where to draw the line' it is clear that several overlapping logics are being mustered into a combined rationale, rather than a single principle or set of empirical facts determining a single cut-off point. What the line is not, or cannot be, thus play as important a role as what it can or might be based on.

Despite its complex rhetorical layering, the poly-logical composition of the 14 day rule is remarkably coherent in retrospect. Its justification is based on a well-ordered set of principles and premises that lead to a simple and unmistakeable series of inter-related and cumulative conclusions. If IVF is permitted, research to improve its safety, efficiency and success must also be permissible. Experiments on embryos must therefore also be permitted. However, given the acute sensitivities and divisions around the issue of human embryo experimentation – and the strong feelings these arouse – a principled compromise is significantly preferable either to no legislation at all or to a patchwork regulatory system. Precisely because of the strength of feeling the subject of human embryo experimentation arouses, both the principles on which the compromise is based, and the regulatory structure developed to enforce it, must be of the very highest integrity. The solution, then, is a highly regulated but permissive apparatus for legislation, backed up by the will of Parliament, and designed to reassure the public and professional communities alike.

Warnock had an even simpler formulation. There was no way, she argued, to definitely determine the moral status of the human embryo: this was a subject on which consensus would never be reached. In contrast, a premise on which almost everyone *could* agree is that legislation of some kind on this issue would be preferable to none. The exact wording of such legislation, she argued, might not seem 'right' to everyone, but if it was 'alright' to enough people, definitive laws and strict regulatory guidelines could replace the 'legal vacuum' surrounding the whole area of assisted reproductive technologies and human embryo research. The alternative would be for the legal vacuum to remain the default – and this 'nobody wants'.

Sticking to this simple maxim was Warnock's guiding compass as she deftly steered away from issues that would either throw her Committee off course or unduly delay them in troubled waters, such as the upper time limit for abortion, instead focussing their attention on the specific questions set out in over 200 detailed briefing papers. To the extent that the 14 day rule is the principled offspring of a polyglot series of compromises, it is nonetheless (or indeed for this very reason) a masterpiece of 'translational' reasoning. Crucially, the rule is based on a highly rigorous interpretation of developmental biology – the sophistication of which is unusually advanced, and at the very cutting edge of scientific research for the time, using terms such as 'toti potency' (sic.) – which had barely even entered specialist scientific journals. Shrewdly, the rule is also based on the sound regulatory principle of being able to count the days on a calendar to determine when a cut-off point is reached. Equally wisely, the rule is based on the moral precept that the legal regulation of highly sensitive areas must be proportionate to their gravity, and hence it is backed up by criminal law. In addition to these elements, the rule is also based on the sociological insight that in order for people to trust in controversial scientific research, it must be subject to the very highest standards of risk assessment, oversight and statutory control. For all of these reasons, the 14 day rule appears not only fair, logical, practical and robust, but also sensible, transparent, enforceable and therefore both 'workable' and trustworthy. All of these distinct strands woven together powerfully affirm Warnock's signature formula as a moral philosopher-cum-legislator, namely that the law ultimately not only enacts, but embodies and represents the 'moral idea of society itself'.

These principles, although differently present in McLaren's thinking, nonetheless informed the style of 'biological reasoning' she brought to the table in the Department of Health's offices, just as they had long informed her work in the lab. The very topic of McLaren's lifelong investigations – the complexity of the formative stages of human biological development – was unusually orientated toward the permeability of these stages to external influences. Her very early experiments on 'uterine effect' explored how the 'outside gets in' and how the 'inside gets out'. In her pursuit of understanding 'everything involved in getting from one generation to the next', McLaren was even more expansive. She considered issues such as the promotion of inclusivity and internationalism in scientific research to be as essential to the production of the very best scientific knowledge as having the latest equipment or technology. She also understood that better science policy required, from the outset, the engagement and involvement of the public at the very heart of the discussions. Scientists were not well served by the assumption that they, by virtue of their training and expertise, automatically knew what was best for society. To the contrary, they should view their role as translators – bringing the public in to science so they could see for themselves its obvious benefits, and taking seriously their responsibility to communicate with non-scientists about their research.

This was exactly what McLaren and Warnock would do from the summer of 1984, when their Report was presented to Parliament, to the enactment of the first Human Fertilisation and Embryology Act six years later, in 1990. Over the six years separating the Warnock Report's publication and the passage of all 64 of the Inquiry's recommendations more or less unchanged into law, a prolonged public and parliamentary debate took place in the UK over IVF, surrogacy, embryo research, and ultimately also over abortion. The most highly contested issue throughout remained the scope of permissible research on human embryos. Inevitably, critics challenged the key distinction on which the regulation was based, between what came to be known as the 'pre-embryo' and the 'embryo proper'. Parliamentary opponents and Right-to-Life activists, joined by MPs, bishops, bioethicists, and some scientists, persistently tried to pick apart the logic of the 14 day rule. For both Mary Warnock and Anne McLaren, the period from 1984 to 1990 was one of almost constant lobbying to enact the Human Fertilisation and Embryology Bill and establish a new Licensing Authority. Ultimately, these became the twin pillars supporting the uniquely 'strict but permissive' climate for human embryonic cell-based experimentation in the UK that has now prevailed for more than three decades.

In practice, this time lag between the publication of the Warnock Report and the enactment of legislation embodying its proposals proved helpful. As McLaren (2004) subsequently explained:

> with hindsight, it was really good to have that 5-year interval before the Human Fertilisation and Embryology Act was passed because there was such a lot of discussion and education and airing of different views during that interval. I think that if there had been any attempt to bring in regulations immediately after the Warnock report, it would not have been so good,

The success of the Warnock Consensus carries valuable lessons regarding the translational process and its relationship to biogovernance generally. Particularly important is its social contract, or formula, of public consultation based on a high degree of trust that the general public will reach a sensible conclusion when they are treated with respect and given time and information to think things through for themselves, combined with a commitment to strict but pragmatic legislative limits.

Among the many lessons the enduring strength of the Warnock Consensus confirms is that controversial bioscientific research can benefit from being publicly debated in highly complex terms, such as the detailed sequences of post-fertilisation development explained in Annex A of Paper 59. Another key lesson from the UK debate over 'developmental landmarks' is that the public can adjust the level of technical detail they want to absorb. This may be particularly important where there are substantial affective dimensions of new biotechniques, such as genome editing, alongside the pragmatic necessity for 'workable' policy and governance. Yet another key legacy of Warnock is the crucial insight that the basis for a good law does not need necessarily to feel 'right' to everyone in order to feel 'alright' to enough people for some legal limits to take the place of none. This means that aiming for a 'combined rationale', rather than seeking a more singular logic, may be a better strategy for reaching consensus on 'sticking points'. Another implication is that 'lines' need not be non-arbitrary in order to be 'workable', and indeed, that lines are employed in arbitration not because they represent certainty but *because they can be changed.*

It may be no coincidence that Mary Warnock and Anne McLaren were both highly successful professionals with somewhat idiosyncratic approaches to their fields who understood and orientated their professional academic lives strongly in terms of public service. They were both also parents and teachers, as well as skilled administrators with excellent communication skills and considerable experience of working on committees. Both were Oxford-educated academics from privileged backgrounds who were known for their ability to take charge of a room when necessary, sometimes with no more than a piercing look. In translating across disciplines and sectors, between different professional communities, and the media, government and the general public, Warnock and McLaren led a process that delivered a remarkable legislative achievement unmatched anywhere since. By laying the foundations for successful national regulation of research on human fertilisation and embryology, in 1983, they delivered proof of principle for a unique system of biogovernance that has now stood for a remarkable length of time.

Conclusion

Although the 14 day rule is in many ways simply a 'line' that establishes a time limit to permissible embryo research, we can see too that both within the legislative architecture of the HFE Bill-then-Act, and in the wider debate surrounding them, the 14 day rule plays another role as a kind of emblem or synecdoche – a part that embodies the whole – for the entire project of governing and regulating 'human fertilisation and embryology'. It is for this reason that the 14 day rule also acts as a kind of condensed signifier of law, science, morality, hope, progress, trust, humanity, society and decency. As we have also seen, the 14 day rule condenses a host of purposes, holding them in a tight arrangement not unlike a secure but complexly interwoven mariner's knot – or perhaps a lengthy tautline hitch. These include the role of law as a binding social force, the moral function and symbolism of regulatory limits, the reciprocal relation between permission and restriction, and the social contract between 'science and society' which is based on trust and exchange. All of these are contextualised by what we might call the long rope of progress and the safety net of the welfare state. Like the 14 day rule, the NHS remains an expressive symbol of reciprocity and mutual care as well as civic obligations. Taking into account the rapid expansion of both the reproductive and regenerative sciences over the past half-century, it is clear that the question of their ongoing translation into future social goods and clinical progress will rely on building inclusive, pragmatic and above all trustworthy foundations of governance and regulation.

Notes

1 Limited polling data suggests that a majority were against public funding for IVF (Beers 2023).
2 In the breakdown by source of correspondence, three categories are identified: (1) 'Letters to [Cabinet] Ministers and the Department' (the DHSS); (2) 'Letters to MPs'; and (3) 'Letters to the Inquiry'. By far the largest single number – 198 (more than twice the total in any other category) – were letters written by constituents to their MPs opposing embryo research.

References

Beers, Laura (2023) 'Not a priority: infertile women and the symbolic politics of IVF in 1980s Britain' *Gender & History* 35(3): 1111–1113.

McLaren, Anne (2004) 'A conversation with Dr Anne McLaren, DBE, DPhil, FRS, FRCOG' *Human Fertility* 7(2): 83–89.

Warnock, Mary (1985) *A question of life: the Warnock Report on human fertilisation and embryology* (Basil Blackwell).

Warnock Committee (1984) *Report of the Committee of Enquiry into Human Fertilisation and Embryology* (HMSO).

Warnock, Mary (2001) 'Anne McLaren as teacher' *The International Journal of Developmental Biology* 45(3): 487–490.

Parliamentary Debates

HL Deb (9 July 1982) vol. 432 cols 1000–1001.

Interviews

Martin Johnson and Sarah Franklin interview with Mary Warnock, Feb. 2008, British Library Oral History Collection.

Martin Johnson and Sarah Franklin interview with Mary Warnock, Feb. 2008, British Library Oral History Collection.

5   The 14 Day Rule since 1990

As we have seen so far, the 14 day rule is both a highly successful regulatory innovation but as the last chapter in particular demonstrates, it is also something of
a chimera – an amalgamation of several layers of reasoning to justify a line being
drawn, when in fact there is not one but several lines that are depicted in various different ways. Famously the system built around this line-that-is-in-fact-several-lines
is at once strict and permissive, firm but flexible, and enduring but adaptable. These
somewhat paradoxical qualities reflect the fundamentally contradictory nature of
the 14 day limit, which is at once arbitrary but not entirely so, and based firmly on
biological facts but also on being able to count to 14. It is also based on the Warnockian principle of being 'if not right at least alright to enough people to enable
some limits rather than none to be established', based in no small part on what
'nobody wants' (i.e. no limits at all).

However, although many of these contradictions have been pointed out as criti-
cisms of the Warnock Report and the 14 day rule, there is, from another point of
view, a clear and purposeful logic uniting them, which we can succinctly describe
as *translational reasoning*. From a translational point of view, it's clear that deploy-
ing many different logics and reasonings, derived from different points of view, is
critical to success. Successful translational reasoning – be it from a strictly biological point of view (in asking how genes receive as well as transmit information for
example) or a legal standard that requires different kinds of proof (biological facts
but also days on a calendar) – by definition has to consider a problem from a wide
range of perspectives. The same is true of insightful sociological analysis and good
policy development, as well as effective communication strategies that build trust
and facilitate effective feedback.

A key concern of this chapter is how the 14 day limit has served as an important
fixed point in the regulatory scheme since 1990, while other aspects of regulation
have come under pressure or strain. The existence of firm limits in the field of human reproduction and embryology has been particularly important given how rapidly this field has developed on several fronts simultaneously. As we saw earlier, it
was always foreseen that basic scientific research into the earliest stages of human
development would continually generate new challenges for the law – many of
which, such as human embryonic stem cell research, somatic cell nuclear transfer
in mammals (cloning), and embryo modelling – have occurred with even greater

DOI: 10.4324/9781003294108-5

speed than either scientists or legislators anticipated in the 1980s. At the same time, human reproduction and embryology have also expanded at breakneck speed clinically and commercially, with the fertility industry now a major sector of the global economy as well as one of the largest areas of private healthcare in the UK. There have also been important social changes, including greater acceptance of a variety of family forms, making access to fertility treatment relevant to more and more people (Golombok 2020).

Here, though, we focus primarily on three crucial legal developments since 1990. First, the statutory purposes for which embryo research could be licensed were extended by Regulations in 2001. Secondly, in 2003, the House of Lords (the UK Supreme Court's predecessor) decided that embryos created using cell nuclear replacement (CNR, the technique used to create Dolly the sheep, and also known as somatic cell nuclear transfer) were embryos for the purposes of the Human Fertilisation and Embryology Act 1990, and were therefore subject to regulation. Thirdly, a major amending piece of primary legislation (the Human Fertilisation and Embryology Act 2008) made substantial changes to the 1990 Act, including specifically bringing human admixed (animal–human hybrid) embryos within regulation.

These changes to the original regulatory regime have, we maintain, crucially relied upon the reassuring certainty that the regulation of embryo research in the UK strictly maintains clear boundaries which are robustly policed by the Human Fertilisation and Embryology Authority – the regulatory body which has overseen the licensing of all research and treatment involving human embryos in the UK since 1991. As an absolute restriction upon what scientists are allowed to do, backed up by tough criminal penalties, the 14 day limit has continuously served a crucial role as the anchor of a robust regulatory system, through which it has been possible to maintain a steady, constant state and yet also to enable continuous evolution and change.

What we are calling 'conditional permissiveness' refers to this combination of strictly maintained conditions that 'back up' or counterbalance the accommodation of new techniques, thus enabling the extension some research horizons (and permitting entirely new ones), while abandoning prohibitions altogether on others (such as donor anonymity and mitochondrial donation). It is by emphasising ongoing compliance with original limitations set out in 1990 that amendments to the original legislation have been facilitated, and new permissions granted on the basis that certain conditions are strictly maintained. Indeed, within this 'strict but permissive' framework, even radically transformative amendments can accurately be depicted as maintaining the principles of the original Act, and the Warnock Report on which it was based. When the research purposes were extended in 2001, for example, legal commentators such as Svea Luise Herrmann (2003) noted that new regulations could be accurately described 'as minimal changes to the existing law that did not entail any new ethical or social implications' due to their compliance with a set of consistent underlying principles. And similarly, when the 2008 amending Bill was before Parliament, biologist Robin Lovell-Badge commented that although the 'HFE Bill incorporates major changes in approach and in the types of research and clinical practice that it will allow ... these are still based on principles that were laid down in the original Act – which the Bill amends rather than replaces – and on the Warnock Report that preceded it' (Lovell-Badge 2008).

Although not named as such in their Report, the principle of 'conditional permissiveness' succinctly captures the basic strategy of the original Warnock proposals for legislation, and in particular the 14 day rule on which they are based. Over time, the enduring success of this strategy has underlined the wisdom of Mary Warnock's early and deliberate decision to sidestep the question of the moral status of the embryo, and to focus instead on how it might be acceptable to treat an early human embryo, the uses to which it might be put, and the limits beyond which such research should not be allowed under any circumstances. This emphasis on acceptable and unacceptable purposes and uses, and clear bright lines dividing them, has played exactly the same pivotal role in facilitating the extension of regulation to encompass new ways of creating and using embryos during the period of rapid bioscientific innovation since the 1990s as it did in enabling the legislation to be passed to begin with (using the 'some limits rather than none' logic). If it had only been possible to discuss what to do about human embryonic stem cell research, somatic cell nuclear replacement and hybrid or admixed embryos by going back to the 'in principle' question of the moral status of the embryo, these discussions would have almost certainly become log-jammed and ultimately derailed by profound and immovable disagreement.

In contrast, and due to the conditional permissiveness principle embodied by the 14 day rule in particular, some (or even significant) adjustment is possible while retaining a steady state of constancy with the original wording and intent of the primary legislation in 1990. Importantly, this principle applies to both permitted and impermissible activities. When the government decided to amend the 1990 Act in the mid-2000s, for example, it made it clear at the outset that certain questions were not open for discussion, one of which was the legality of embryo research (Herrmann 2003). Similarly, when the HFEA consulted on the regulation of hybrid embryos in 2007, it stated firmly that it was not reopening the question of the legality of their creation. Carrying out public consultations while ruling out consideration of certain questions has, of course, been criticised by those who consider this sort of consultation tokenistic, undertaken only in order to comply with political obligations, or 'strategic', and just intended to persuade the public of the merits of the preferred policy option (Baylis 2009). An alternative view, and one we share, is that setting clear parameters to public debate, as well as consultation, can improve their quality by more precisely defining their focus. If a total ban on IVF and embryo research is not politically realistic, public consultation which becomes side-tracked by intractable disagreement on whether IVF and embryo research should be permitted at all will not facilitate genuine public input into whatever new limits are under discussion.

Relying on precedent to limit the scope of debate also builds trust, by facilitating constructive dialogue and established points of consensus rather than polarisation around issues that have already been resolved and do not need to be revisited. The continuity and stability provided by this model of iterative and additive change also promotes a more conducive environment for translational work, and this has been especially important for translational bioscience as IVF and embryo research have greatly expanded over the past three decades. Indeed, an exceptional and unique feature of the biotranslational environment in the UK is its highly regulated but permissive stance toward research on human embryos. Since 1990, the question of the permissibility of embryo research has not been substantively reopened, and the maintenance of this position has strong public support. The most recent figures, from 2022 confirm widespread public support for both embryo research and the 14 day rule (Progress Educational Trust, 2022). We are among many commentators, including the political scientists Shelia Jasanoff and Ingrid Metzler cited in our Introduction, who maintain that the existence of the 14 day limit is a significant factor, along with the reputation of the regulator, that has made it easier to strike out from consideration the question of whether embryo research should be allowed at all. Indeed, using language very similar to our own definition of 'conditional permissiveness', the HFEA suggested in a 2005 newsletter on the proposed creation of hybrid embryos that 'the legislative framework should be broadly permissive [of such research] *on the condition that this remains within the 14 day limit*' (quoted in Baylis 2009, our emphasis).

Notably, this perception of a 'virtuous circle' whereby firm legislation around embryo research facilitates greater public confidence and thus a more beneficial environment for translational bioscience is seen by many to contain a larger message for science policy as it affects issues such as regenerative medicine, and the use of new techniques such as gene editing. In parliamentary debates over sequential changes to the Act, for example, a common refrain is how tough the UK's regulatory regime is, and how well it works. In 2002, for example, the House of Lords Select Committee on Stem Cell Research found that:

> The regulatory system established by the 1990 Act has worked well. The lynchpin of the system is the HFEA. Its work is highly regarded, both at home and abroad. It appeared from the evidence we received that it has the full confidence of the scientific and medical research community, and we believe that it has also been instrumental in reassuring the public that regulation in a particularly emotive area of public policy is carried out effectively and sensitively. It is striking that there have been few legal challenges to the HFEA's rulings and that media criticism has often been on the ground that the Authority is too strict rather than too lax.
>
> (House of Lords 2002: para 8.1)

Adding to the chorus, Dame Suzi Leather, then Chair of the HFEA, told the House of Commons Science and Technology Select Committee in 2004 that the UK has 'a quieter environment, in a sense, for the cutting edge research, embryonic stem cell research, in this country than, for instance, in the United States', and that 'some of that can be put down to regulation' (House of Commons 2004: para. 356). Similarly, in her evidence to the House of Commons Science and Technology Committee in 2007, Anne McLaren told the Committee that the UK has a 'sensible and scientifically-based regulatory system that has functioned with few major problems for the past 16 years' (House of Commons 2004: para. 18). The BioIndustry Association further informed the Committee that 'in the HFEA, the UK has a world class regulator', and it argued for the continuance of a 'robust regulatory system that inspires public confidence and is supportive of groundbreaking medical research' (ibid.: para. 64).

This system of 'tough but permissive' regulation has been supported by philosophers and scientists as well as legislators and parliamentarians. For example, philosopher Onora O'Neill (2003) says she has 'come to have great respect for the drafters of the 1990 Human Fertilisation and Embryology Act', because they have produced 'a system of regulation of embryo research with a clear default structure', and she goes on to note, that '[a]s the statistics show, licenses have been sparingly granted'. Scientists too have praised the role of firm barriers in building public confidence. For example, Robin Lovell-Badge points out that:

> UK scientists on the whole feel comfortable knowing precisely where the barriers are, and have the benefit of both government support and a public that has been reassured that any work has been thoroughly assessed before being allowed to proceed.
>
> (Lovell-Badge 2008)

Indeed, time and again since 1990, UK laws governing human fertilisation and embryology have been enabled to become more permissive precisely by emphasising the strictness, efficiency and transparency of the UK's regulatory regime. As Herrmann (2003) puts it, 'the emphasis on limitation and control [has] served as an important pro-research argument'. In the process of essentially loosening restrictions on embryo research, 'the assurance that research was subject to control and limitation was decisive ... leading to the apparent paradox of deregulation via regulation'. As noted earlier, however, this paradox is in many ways both a logical outcome of a broadly inclusive and wide-ranging process of translational reasoning and a feature of the inherently iterative, interdisciplinary and multifaceted translational process itself, which by definition has to include perspectives from all angles while remaining tightly focussed on a specific goal.

Neutralising 'Moral Status' Arguments

As we consider in more depth the distinctive role the 14 day limit has played in creating a stable and conducive climate for biotranslational science in the UK, and the importance (or not) of 'conditional permissiveness' to this process, it is helpful to examine three key moments in the 2000s when liberalising changes were introduced, and to look at how, exactly, these were implemented. In turn we can better understand both the claim that the 14 day limit is an enabler of liberalisation, and how it has come to function as a symbol as well as a means of promoting public trust in scientific research.

As noted earlier, during the first parliamentary debates on embryo research immediately following the publication of the Warnock Report in 1984, and while the

Human Fertilisation and Embryology Bill was being debated five years later in the 1989–90 parliamentary session, concern for the moral status of the embryo was much more prominently and vigorously articulated from many different quarters than it is today. With some notable exceptions – such as Sir Trevor Skeet MP who said that infertility 'can cause no greater anguish than the lot of a very plain girl who fails to marry' (HC Deb 4 February 1988) – there was considerable sympathy for the plight of infertile couples. But it was repeatedly argued that however severe this anguish might be, it had to be balanced against the unique degree of respect due to the human embryo. For example, Tony Newton MP claimed that if 'due respect must be given in law to the presence of human life [then] unequivocally ... the early embryo must be protected in law', and he similarly drew attention to the tension 'between the need to protect the early embryo and the need to offer as much help as possible to infertile couples' (HC Deb 4 February 1988). In the House of Lords, Lord Skelmersdale noted that 'research using human embryos can bring great benefits. However, the human embryo deserves respect and the protection of the law', before asking '[h]ow complete should that protection be?' (HL Deb 15 January 1988).

As noted earlier, the Warnock Committee's decision to shift the fundamental question it asked itself about research on the early human embryo from 'what is its moral status?' to 'how can it be treated?' has had far reaching consequences, most of which have been overwhelmingly positive for science and scientific progress. There was, however, considerable and well-organised opposition to this approach in Parliament. For example, Sir Bernard Braine MP, head of the Cross-Party Parliamentary Pro-Life Committee, demanded to know why 'instead of trying to answer the [moral status] questions directly we have therefore gone straight to the question of how it is right to treat the human embryo', and described it as 'odd' that the Warnock Committee would even consider addressing the question of how to treat the human embryo 'without being clear about what it really was'.

Although the Warnock Report was clear that the embryo had a 'special status', it did not try to define exactly what this is, and instead turned to the practical questions of what could legitimately be done with it, within what limits. In addition to shifting the focus away from intractable arguments about the moral status of the embryo, and the related controversy about abortion, this approach also put great emphasis on the essential relationship between IVF and embryo research. Since allowing treatments such as IVF would require corresponding investment in embryo research, this research was directly linked to the relief of human suffering. The emphasis on embryo research also refocussed attention on disease prevention via the newly possible and near horizon technique of PGT.[1] Connecting the human embryo to embryology, and embryo research to improved fertility treatment and the possibility of preventing genetic disease not only offered a concrete set of tangible social goods, but enabled the Committee to focus upon practical questions about permissible use. The abstract onto-theological question of the human embryo's moral status became both plural (which embryos?) and pragmatic (for which purposes are they being used), as well as contextual (where and by whom are they being put to use). These shifts in turn focused minds on the question of what are or are not morally acceptable ways to treat the human embryo, rather than returning to first principles and considering whether any instrumental use of human embryos is compatible with their moral status.

Although strategically defensive, and initially mobilised in the face of considerable opposition to human embryo research – by a well-organised Pro-Life movement with many influential parliamentary representatives, and a generally conservative political climate – the shift of debate toward permissible uses of embryos rather than their status 'in principle' has proven both popular and effective. Coupled with the introduction of the 14 day rule, the emphasis on allowing strictly limited research within rigorously enforced limits, overseen by a designated Authority, both enabled an inclusive compromise and established a robust regulatory platform that could endure over time. As John Gillott has explained, this innovative regulatory infrastructure enabled the UK to move 'from a framework centered on respecting the "special status" of the human embryo to one that includes this within a process-orientated governance framework' (Gillott 2013). This was and remains a unique accomplishment unmatched by any other country or legislature and has rightly been described as both an ingenious and inclusive means of governing bioscience.

Although possibly for tactical reasons, it has become less common to hear opposition to embryo research grounded in the sanctity of embryonic human life,[2] and the rapid normalisation of IVF has significantly weakened the popular purchase of anti-embryo research arguments.[3] More commonly, concerns are expressed about slippery slopes (Gillott 2013); 'touchpaper' issues such as 'designer babies' and cloning; the potential for exploitation of gamete donors and surrogates; and commercialisation (Deech 2002).

The question of how much respect is due to the early human embryo has been largely absent from parliamentary debates on embryo research since 1990. Indeed, during the early 2000s when Parliament first discussed the possibility of extending the permissible purposes for which embryo research could be carried out, even these extensions' opponents instead relied upon essentially utilitarian arguments, by disputing whether embryo research was in fact beneficial and/or necessary – and thus by default confirming the default criteria of permissible and impermissible purposes. Thus, when the Roman Catholic MP Ruth Kelly claimed in 2000 in opposition to embryo research that 'it is difficult to point to any real advances in the treatment of congenital diseases that have been made as a result of the research' (HC Deb 15 December 2000), she also revealed her (perhaps pragmatic) reluctance any longer to use faith-based arguments to support her case in Parliament. Research involving adult stem cells was also cited in order to claim that it was now no longer necessary to use embryos in research. Likewise, when Tory MP Bill Cash, who has repeatedly sought to restrict abortion law since 1984, claimed in a 2008 parliamentary debate that he was 'not suggesting that we should stop all [embryo] research' but that 'we have alternatives such as adult stem-cell research' that should be used instead, he was somewhat ironically confirming exactly why a more progressive set of laws governing research are needed (HC Deb 19 May 2008).

Rebutting 'Slippery Slope' Claims

Although the 14 day rule has been instrumental in helping to maintain the emphasis on permissible and impermissible uses of embryos, rather than their moral status, and this in turn has enabled the 'process-orientated governance structure' described by John Gillott above, the use of a time limit has also been a frequent target of critics who question its fitness for purpose. In particular, opponents of embryo research have long made liberal use of the 'slippery slope' argument that limits can be changed. A related argument holds that rogue scientists could ignore such limits entirely. During the early parliamentary debates in the 1980s, there were frequent accounts in both the popular press and on the floor of Parliament detailing the horrors that might be unleashed through illicit research on human embryos. In the very first discussion of the Warnock Report in the House of Lords following its publication in 1984, the Eton and Oxford educated Lord Ian Maitland, the 18th Earl of Lauderdale, expressed his grave concerns about 'the virtual manufacture of children before even birth, denied the security of identifiable parents in homes of compassion and care' as well as 'the possibility of genetic manipulation to breed, for example – rather like Japanese bonsai trees – a race of tiny persons for high altitude flying and space travel' (HL Deb 31 October 1984).

In the same parliamentary session, the Conservative Peer Lord Coleraine was concerned that 14 days was less an iron-clad limit than a brazen stalking horse designed to secure a 'foot in the door' – and thus 'an open invitation' to keep embryos alive indefinitely:

> Is it not apparent that the majority favour a much longer period for experimentation, and view 14 days as the most that public opinion can be persuaded to accept at this moment, and at the same time regard it as the necessary foot in the door, opening it in fact if not in law to unlimited research? That is what it would prove to be – an open invitation to pass through an open door. It might be difficult to police a total ban on the creation and keeping alive of human embryos for purposes other than implantation. It would be well-nigh impossible to monitor the work of research scientists to ensure that they do not exceed a 14-days' maximum.
>
> (HL Deb 31 October 1984)

A month later, Jill Knight MP flatly denied scientists could be kept in check: 'Would the scientists really down scalpels [sic] at 11.55 pm on the 14th day? Of course not' (HC Deb 23 November 1984).

The likelihood that the 14 day limit would be breached emerged as a common theme throughout the debates. In a later debate in the House of Commons as the Bill began its final passage into law, Mary Warnock's comment in an interview that the 14 day limit 'would do for a start' was seized upon by MPs who opposed embryo research as evidence that, as Sir Bernard Braine MP, leader of the All-Party Pro-Life group, alleged, the slide had already begun: 'We are on a downward slide with these people and we do not know where it will end', he claimed in open debate on the floor of the House of Commons (HC Deb 4 February 1988). In the same debate, the barrister Sir Trevor Skeet, a Tory MP, asked what would prevent the limit being extended to more than a month, thus enabling the pursuit of a master race, as envisioned by Hitler:

> Why have a limit of 14 days? Why should it not be extended to 20, 30 or 40 days? The ultimate goal may be to produce a child entirely *in vitro* or to produce genetically identical individuals by cloning. In other words, the goal may be to mimic the natural process leading to selective breeding or the creation of human beings with predetermined characteristics. Those of us of my generation will recognise exactly what Hitler did and we remember his domination and his concept of the master race. One can see that coming, not in a lifetime but in two lifetimes.
>
> (HC Deb 4 February 1988)

In one of the final debates on the HFE Bill, in April 1990, just prior to its passage into law, Skeet once again voiced his scepticism about whether 14 days would 'hold':

> It is all very well the Secretary of State alleging that he will keep to 14 days. We know that 14 days will be breached at the first opportunity, as soon as it can be established that there is more material gain to be secured thereafter. Fourteen days is not immutable.
>
> (HC Deb 23 April 1990)

In the same debate, Sir Michael McNair-Wilson MP asked 'how soon will it be before we are told that, if only we could have another 14 days, they could achieve so much more?' (HC Deb 23 April 1990). Similarly, Patrick Duffy MP was sceptical of the claim that 'the 14-day limit represents such a significant break point in human development that it will act as an anchor and prevent any drift beyond the agreed limit', asking 'How many hon Members share such optimism?' Citing with concern Bob Edwards' comment that embryology 'is a gradual process of steady change', he went on to say 'I suspect that some hon Members would support research if they could be sure that it would be strictly controlled' (HC Deb 23 April 1990). When the Bill had been debated in the House of Lords, the Lord Bishop of London had also expressed the fear that the 14 day limit would be unlikely to last: 'before too long we shall have legislation extending the 14-day period. Such developments have been stated in regard to previous legislation. I am trying to be realistic' (HL Deb 4 February 1990).

Other members of the House of Lords were more confident that clear statutory limits would prevent a slide down the slope. For example, Lord Bridge of Harwich (who was also a member of the House of Lords Judicial Committee, the UK Supreme Court's predecessor) said that:

> The answer to the slippery slope argument to my mind is found in Chapter 11 of the report of the committee of the noble Baroness, which indicates

perfectly valid, pragmatic reasons for choosing a biologically sensible and defensible cut-off point ... When this Bill becomes an Act of Parliament, that cut-off point will be given Parliamentary sanction in the form of the provisions of Clause 3 and it will be given the sanction of the law. Once it has that sanction, I simply do not understand why it is said that it will be difficult to maintain the cut-off point. It can and should be maintained.

(HL Deb 4 February 1990)

Viscount Caldecote was similarly reassured by the 14 day limit:

there is a break point at 14 days. That it is not the start of running down a slippery slope. There is a real step in that slope which will prevent us going further down it if we have any sense. I am therefore not worried about that aspect.

(HL Deb 7 December 1989)

In 1989–1990, therefore, although the majority voted in favour of legislation to permit embryo research within the 14 day limit, a significant minority was concerned that it was unlikely to work as a bulwark against the slippery slope.

When the question of embryo research returned to Parliament a decade later, in the context of a possible extension of the purposes for which embryo research could be licensed, parliamentarians instead emphasised the reassurance offered by the 14 day limit, and concerns that it might be exceeded had effectively been silenced. Indeed, by 2000, the 14 day limit had become a principal reason to be *confident* in the strictness of the regulation of embryo research. Then Parliamentary Under-Secretary of State for Public Health, Yvette Cooper MP said:

Under the 1990 Act, no research can take place beyond 14 days. The Government do not advocate any research beyond that point, as it is not appropriate. The safeguards in the Act are clear. A separate issue is understanding the development of cells – cells not embryos – extracted from embryos. It is important to understand how they develop, but it is important that any research does not involve embryos beyond 14 days. That is clear in the Act and the regulations.

(HC Deb 19 December 2000)

Of course, an important difference in 2000 compared with 1989–90 is that there was, by then, evidence of how the Act and the HFEA had worked in practice for nearly a decade. Dr Ian Gibson MP pointed to evidence that the 14 day limit had held, and he was confident it would continue to do so:

In the 10 years since 1990, no problems have arisen with research licences. No breaches of the 1990 Act have occurred and no scientists have conducted unlicensed research. Many people are suspicious of the arrogance of science and so on, but every centre is inspected annually, the research community is closely knit, there is strong professionalism and control is tight. I doubt

whether anybody would be tempted to go beyond the use of a 14-day embryo merely for the sake of kudos in the scientific community. Such a person would be jumped on heavily and his or her professionalism would be
destroyed.

(HC Deb 15 December 2000)

Facilitating Arguments about the Importance of Science/Innovation for the UK Economy

Since 1990, as well as hearing much less about the sanctity of human embryonic
life, it has become increasingly common for discussion of the regulation of embryo research to raise as a relevant consideration the impact of regulation on UK
science, and UK plc (House of Commons 2007: para 103). When emergency legislation to ban human reproductive cloning was debated, Dr Desmond Turner MP
commented that:

> We are fortunate that we have established a sensible regulatory regime for
> work on embryos. Medical scientists in this country know the boundaries.
> They know what they can and cannot do and that as long as they work within
> them, they are safe from attack. That is not the case in the rest of Europe
> where medical scientists feel unsafe and are disinclined to work in the field.
> This country benefits from taking a lead in such research.
>
> (HC Deb 29 November 2001)

In particular, supporters of embryo research argue that its tough-yet-permissive
system of regulation enables UK science to 'punch above its weight'. This then
becomes a compelling argument for liberalising amendments, because to fail to
support them is to harm UK science, and by extension the UK economy.

When the research purposes were extended, those who supported the extension
relied upon 'the necessity of scientific progress for the improvement of British society, economy and international competitiveness', and expressed concerns about
'a possible 'brain drain' and thus the potential loss of Britain's standing at the
forefront of international biotechnology' (Herrmann 2003). For example, Baroness
Warwick of Undercliffe said that any delay in passing the Regulations would:

> mean that our scientists in universities and in industry would lose any hope
> of remaining at the cutting edge of the technology which involves a branch
> of science in which the UK is currently pre-eminent.
>
> (HL Deb 22 January 2001)

In its review of the Human Fertilisation and Embryology Act 1990 in the mid-2000s,
the House of Commons Science and Technology Select Committee heard from scientists that the current system is 'the single most important reason why we have
taken a lead worldwide in stem cell research', and that the HFEA 'is a huge part
of the engine that drives forward stem cell research' (2004, para 341). Ruth Deech
(2002), who was Chair of the HFEA from 1994 to 2002, has said that '[i]n Britain

we believe we are ahead of the field, not only in the quality of research but in its public acceptability and respectability. This is, we believe, due to the legislation and the tight regulation'.

Two years later, in responding to the government's proposed ban on the creation of hybrid embryos, the Science and Technology Select Committee (2007) again stressed the importance of considering the impact of regulation on UK science:

> the UK's regulatory system has traditionally been viewed as an important element in the pre-eminency of the UK in this scientific field. It has been viewed with envy by researchers from countries with more restrictive regimes and it has been influential in the development of policy-making in other countries. There have to be concerns that changes to the regulatory system should not harm the reputation and make-up of the UK science base but should encourage it to develop in order to realise the expectations placed on it in terms of knowledge and tackling disease.
>
> (Science and Technology Select Committee 2007: para 103)

As we see below, the government was initially reluctant to permit the creation of human-animal hybrid embryos, and this reluctance was fiercely criticised by the Science and Technology Select Committee:

> A ban and the prospect of a ban in draft legislation on human-animal chimera or hybrid embryos would undermine the UK's leading position in stem cell research and the international reputation of science in the UK.
>
> (Science and Technology Select Committee 2007: para 104)

The UK was said to have a 'competitive advantage' in stem cell research, which the government's proposed ban would eliminate:

> We are concerned that a ban or a proposed ban may not only encourage researchers to leave the UK in order to undertake their research in a more permissive regulatory regime, but it may also inhibit early stage researchers entering the field. Whilst we do not believe that UK competitiveness should dictate policy in a research area, we believe that the Government should consider this as a contributory factor and we recommend that the Government ensure that it is properly briefed on potential implications from future legislation in this area.
>
> (Science and Technology Select Committee 2007: para 107)

Commenting on the new boundaries set by the 2008 amending Bill, Robin Lovell-Badge (2008) said that he was 'content that the boundaries will have been expanded sufficiently to allow new, exciting research, and to help keep the United Kingdom competitive', while at the same time warning that:

> this and future governments need to retain the close links with scientists and to act fast when the need arises: there will continue to be advances, some

from the United Kingdom, but many from other countries without the same regulatory constraints.

(Lovell-Badge 2008)

True to Lovell-Badge's prediction, the past 15 years have indeed seen very rapid changes within both scientific research and fertility treatment. At the same time, and largely due to its robust regulatory structure, the UK has been able to lead in both biomedical research as well as adapting its regulatory environment and science policy. Indeed, as we saw earlier, one characteristic of the UK's regulatory environment is that it has enabled the approval of new processes and the creation of new entities, without at the same time producing moral panics or political stand-offs. Three of these changes are especially relevant to the question of the 14 day rule: extending the research purposes to include stem cell research, cell nuclear replacement and the creation of human admixed embryos.

Stem Cell Research

In addition to complying with the 14 day limit, and establishing that the use of embryos in research is necessary (that is, the research could not be carried out using animals or adult cells), the HFEA can only grant a research licence if the proposed research is 'necessary or desirable' for one of the statutory purposes. Specifying the purposes for which research on embryos can be carried out is another restriction which is intended to provide public reassurance that this sort of research is very tightly controlled, and directed towards self-evidently valuable ends.

The original purposes, set out in Schedule 2(3)(2) of the Act, were:

(a)   promoting advances in the treatment of infertility,
(b)   increasing knowledge about the causes of congenital disease,
(c)   increasing knowledge about the causes of miscarriage,
(d)   developing more effective techniques of contraception, or
(e)   developing methods for detecting the presence of gene or chromosome abnormalities in embryos before implantation,

or for such other purposes as may be specified in regulations. (our emphasis)

This last italicised sentence is an attempt to 'future-proof' the legislation, in case unanticipated research purposes subsequently emerged. It was used for the first time in 2001, in order to accommodate the use of human embryos in stem cell research.

In 1998, researchers at the University of Wisconsin published a paper explaining how they had, for the first time, derived and cultured a human embryonic stem cell line (Thomson et al. 1998). This was ground-breaking research, because the inner cell mass of the early human embryo contains stem cells of remarkable plasticity. Not only can they become every cell in the human body, but they are also immortal, and can continue to divide indefinitely without losing their genetic structure. More remarkably still, it was thought that if stem cells could be extracted from CNR embryos, the tissue generated would be genetically identical to the donor of the adult cell used to create a bespoke immortal cell line that could be used to replace damaged tissue or repair malfunctioning organs such as the heart, pancreas or liver. If this technique, which became known as 'therapeutic cloning', could be perfected, it was thought that it might be capable of eliminating the problem of rejection in tissue transplantation, as well as eradicating the shortage of donor tissues and organs.

Following this announcement, in 1998 the HFEA and the since disbanded Human Genetics Advisory Commission undertook a major public consultation on human cloning and stem cell research. Their report recommended that new regulations should extend the purposes for which embryo research could be carried out in the UK. The government then set up an expert group, chaired by the Chief Medical Officer (CMO) Professor Sir Liam Donaldson, to assess the possible benefits of stem cell research, and to further advise whether regulations should extend the purposes for which the HFEA might issue licences for research involving human embryos. In 2000, the CMO's Expert Group's report agreed that the potential benefits of this sort of research justified the use of human embryos as a source of stem cells. It also recommended that before licensing any human embryonic stem cell (hESC) research project, the HFEA should satisfy itself that there are no other means of meeting the objectives of the research, and that individuals whose eggs or sperm are used to create the embryos to be used in research should give specific consent to their use in a research project to derive stem cells.

Following the CMO's Expert Group's endorsement of hESC research, the government brought forward Regulations extending the purposes for which research on human embryos could be lawfully undertaken. Schedule 2's additional research purposes are intended to accommodate stem cell research into the treatment of serious medical conditions, as well as basic research:

(a) increasing knowledge about serious disease or other serious medical conditions,

(b) developing treatments for serious disease or other serious medical conditions,

(c) increasing knowledge about the causes of any congenital disease or congenital medical condition that does not fall within paragraph (a) …

(d) increasing knowledge about the development of embryos.

In the parliamentary debates on these Regulations, Svea Luise Herrmann (2003) draws attention to the emphasis placed on 'the importance of embryonic stem cell research for society and for the individual sufferer of "serious diseases"'. The clear establishment of a connection between innovative biomedical research and a translational purpose could be expressed as fulfilling 'a need within society', she points out, producing 'a strong moralising effect'. This view was clearly evident in parliamentary debate. For example, introducing the Regulations in the House of Lords,

Parliamentary Under-Secretary of State Lord Hunt of Kings Heath explained the future benefits of embryonic stem cell research:

> We shall learn how to manipulate the cells from our own bodies to produce the tissues that we need, whether for our heart should we develop heart failure, or brain tissue for Parkinson's, or nervous tissue for our spines should we become paralysed in an accident. That is the ultimate aim for which the proposed embryo research is one temporary step along the journey... I doubt that there is a single person or family who has not been touched at some time by the distress that some of those diseases bring. It is said that more than half of the world's diseases have no effective treatment and that we are unable to develop drugs, or other treatments to cure or alleviate many of those conditions. In any case, drugs are not always the answer, and never will be. In these cases, the only treatment that is likely to offer chance of a real cure is one based on the person's own body, a treatment which is cell-based and individual.
>
> (HL Deb 22 January 2001)

Contrasts were also drawn with the existing research purposes. As Under-Secretary of State Yvette Cooper MP put it:

> If embryo research on infertility is acceptable, surely research for Parkinson's disease should be too? If embryo research for contraception is acceptable, surely research for muscular dystrophy should be too?
>
> (HC Deb 19 December 2000)

Although the Regulations were passed, there was some disquiet about dealing with a matter of this importance through unamendable Regulations. As Pro-Life former MP Lord Alton explained:

> It is wholly inappropriate to use unamendable regulations to deal with an issue of this importance... I add that this is a curiously convoluted world in which we can find parliamentary time for a Bill that protects foxes but we cannot find time for a Bill that will lead to the manufacture and elimination of countless human embryos. Regulations of this kind also dispense with the dreary business of detailed scrutiny, transparency and proper parliamentary opposition. The danger of dispensing with due process is that democracy will be brought into disrepute and that public cynicism about our institutions will simply be deepened. That is why, along with noble Lords with whom I differ on the status of the human embryo, such as my noble friend Lady Warnock and the right reverend Prelate the Bishop of Oxford, we have offered an alternative today that will allow for sober reflection and for proper debate.
>
> (HL Deb 22 January 2001)

An amendment was therefore passed in order to appoint a Select Committee 'to consider and report on the issues connected with human cloning and stem cell research arising from the Human Fertilisation and Embryology (Research Purposes) Regulations'. Setting up a Select Committee after rather than before legislative reform is unusual. Because of the contentiousness of the issue, the HFEA chose not to issue any licences under the new Regulations until the House of Lords Select Committee had concluded its deliberations.

Once established, the Select Committee (2002) decided to take 'a fresh look at those aspects of [the Warnock] report relevant to our remit', including 'the fundamental question of the status of the embryo' and 'the creation of embryos for research, an issue on which the Warnock Committee was divided' (para 1.17). This 'fresh look' did not result in any deviation from the Warnock approach, however:

> Whilst respecting the deeply held views of those who regard any research involving the destruction of a human embryo as wrong and having weighed the ethical arguments carefully, the Committee is not persuaded, especially in the context of the current law and social attitudes, that all research on early human embryos should be prohibited.
>
> (House of Lords 2002: para 4.21)

In the light of the Select Committee's approval of human embryonic stem cell research, the first licences were granted soon afterwards by the HFEA, and within two years, one-third of the 30 research projects licensed in the UK involved hESC research (HFEA 2004).

Although it supported the extension of the research purposes, the House of Lords Select Committee did suggest that it might be helpful for the HFEA to undertake a review of the outcomes from embryo research projects, on the grounds that the 'public is entitled to know whether the claims made for human embryo research have been realised'. The Committee also drew attention to the fact that 'therapeutic cloning' would require a continuing supply of human eggs, from which the nucleus could be removed.

Egg donation is uncomfortable and invasive, and not entirely risk-free. Given that there is a shortage of donor eggs for use in fertility treatment, there was unlikely to be an endless supply of human eggs available for stem cell research. Moreover, at the time of the HL Report, in 2002, the process of deriving stem cell lines from human embryos was at an early stage with unpredictable success rates. Some scientists therefore argued that it would be foolish, or even unethical, to use scarce human eggs to perfect these techniques. Following a major scandal in 2004 involving a South Korean researcher, Hwang Woo-suk, who was found to have conducted fraudulent research allegedly involving hundreds of donated eggs from female volunteers, concerns about the sources of donor ova for research purposes was heightened.[4] In 2006 the Yamanaka lab at Kyoto University revealed a simple new method to 'induce' pluripotent (embryo-like) stem cells from adult (differentiated) mouse cells, and to create immortalised cell lines from this source instead of embryos. In 2007 they repeated this work using human cells. This work underscored the importance of continuing to pursue basic research on animal eggs, including material retrieved from abattoirs, which could be readily obtained in large numbers. As Robin Lovell-Badge explained:

> Donated human eggs are in short supply, especially for research. If animal eggs do work, it was felt ethically unsound to put women through the procedures that are required to obtain eggs, especially when the cloning methods are so inefficient.
>
> (Lovell-Badge 2008)

These and other developments, including the use of transgenic human-animal cells for the purpose of cloning livestock who could produce human proteins in their milk, led to the third extension to the original statutory scheme which we consider below: the creation of certain sorts of animal-human hybrid embryos, referred to in legislation as human admixed embryos.

Cell Nuclear Replacement

The announcement in 1997 that an adult sheep had been successfully cloned through CNR created difficulties for regulation, because of an unfortunately worded subsection in the 1990 Act. Dolly the sheep had been created by removing the nucleus from a sheep's egg, and inserting a cell from an adult sheep into the denucleated egg (Wilmut et al. 1997). Using an electric current, this egg was then 'quickened' into beginning the process of cell division. This process led to the creation of a sheep embryo, and to the birth of a sheep, but it did not involve fertilisation. Since the original section 1(1)(a) of the 1990 Act stated: 'In this Act ... embryo means a live human embryo where fertilisation is complete', the question arose whether an embryo created using CNR, also known as somatic cell nuclear transfer, is an embryo for the purposes of regulation.

This potential gap in the statutory scheme did not arise because the drafters of the 1990 legislation had failed to anticipate the possibility of mammalian or human cloning. Rather, they had assumed that cloning for this purpose would only be possible if *fertilised* eggs were used, in which case any cloned human embryos would fall within the 'definition' in section 1, and their creation would amount to a criminal offence via section 3(3)(d) of the Act (which prohibits 'replacing a nucleus of a cell of an embryo with a nucleus taken from a cell of any person, embryo or subsequent development of an embryo').

The apparent gap between the statutory wording and the procedure involved in Dolly's creation was the subject of a judicial review action brought by Bruno Quintavalle, on behalf of the Pro-life Alliance. Mr Quintavalle claimed that the definition of 'embryo' in the 1990 Act did not cover embryos created by CNR. The implications of this would be extremely serious. The Act makes it a criminal offence to produce an embryo outside of a woman's body except in pursuance of a licence granted by the HFEA. But if a cloned embryo is not an embryo for the purposes of the Act, cloning is not a licensable activity, and would therefore be subject to no statutory restrictions at all. If they were unregulated, cloned 'embryos' could be produced without any oversight, meaning that they could be cultured *in vitro* well beyond 14 days and even transferred to a woman's uterus.

Of course, Mr Quintavalle was not the first person to notice the lack of fit between section 1 of the Human Fertilisation and Embryology Act and CNR, but it had been assumed that because it was so plainly Parliament's intention that all embryos should fall within the regulatory framework, a purposive interpretation of these words would be sufficient to bring CNR embryos within the HFEA's licensing regime (Plomer 2002). At first instance, however, Mr Quintavalle succeeded. The government had argued that the subsection should be read as if it read: 'a live human embryo where [if it is produced by fertilisation] fertilisation is complete', but Crane J held that the words in the statute were not sufficiently ambiguous to allow him to ignore their clear meaning.

Following Crane J's judgment, cloning was therefore unregulated in the UK. This was not Mr Quintavalle's preferred outcome. Rather he wanted Parliament to revisit the regulation of embryo research, with the hope that this would result in more restrictive legislation. In the immediate aftermath of Crane J's judgment, emergency legislation was passed to ban reproductive cloning. Crane J's judgment was subsequently reversed by the Court of Appeal, and the House of Lords dismissed Mr Quintavalle's appeal.

There was a difference between the Court of Appeal and the House of Lords' judgments in *Quintavalle*. The Court of Appeal's view was that it was of such importance that all embryos are covered by the legislation, that this must have been what Parliament had intended. A strained interpretation of the statutory language was therefore permissible in order to uphold Parliament's clear and unambiguous intention. In contrast, in dismissing Mr Quintavalle's appeal, the House of Lords did not admit to having had to strain the language in the statute. Instead, it held that 'embryo' is an ordinary word of the English language—and that cloned embryos are undoubtedly embryos. Section 1(1)(a) was not intended to offer a special statutory redefinition of the word 'embryo'. Rather the normal meaning of the word embryo must have been taken for granted by parliamentary counsel (who are responsible for drafting legislation) because the definition is 'a live human embryo where fertilisation is complete'. This 'definition' contains the word it is supposed to define, with no further elaboration. The important words in this phrase, according to Lord Millett, are therefore 'live' and 'human'— this is the *sort* of embryo that is regulated by the statute—so dead and animal embryos are not covered.

The House of Lords also appeared to be assisted by looking at what Parliament did *not* intend when passing section 1(1)(a). Its purpose, they argued, was not to distinguish between different ways in which embryos might be created, because at that time it did not occur to anyone that they could be created unless an egg had been fertilised. Hence the phrase 'when fertilisation is complete' was intended to identify *when* an embryo would be subject to regulatory control, and not the manner in which the embryo had been created.

Of course, it could be argued that it is not strictly true to say that Parliament did not anticipate cloning, and did not have any intention about how such embryos should be regulated, since section 3(3)(d) does attempt to ban the only sort of cloning which it was believed might become feasible. In any event, the reforms to the 1990 Act effected by the 2008 amending statute removed the reference to fertilisation in section 1, which now reads: 'In this Act . . . embryo means a live human embryo and does not include a human admixed embryo'.

As a result of the House of Lords' decision in *Quintavalle*, it was clear that the HFEA had the power to issue licences for the creation of human embryos using CNR for research purposes. The researchers who received the first CNR licence in August 2004 announced the following year that they had successfully cloned four human embryos, one of which was successfully cultured for five days (Stojkovic 2005).

Human Admixed Embryos

The 1990 Act has always permitted one very narrowly circumscribed combination of animal and human gametes, through what was known as the 'zona-free hamster-egg test', which involved testing the fertility of human sperm using hamster eggs, and destroying any resulting 'embryo' no later than the two-cell stage. In practice, the hamster test is no longer in regular use, in part due to its limited accuracy, and in part because of the development of techniques like intracytoplasmic sperm injection (ICSI).

The use of animal material in basic embryonic stem cell research was first mooted towards the end of the twentieth century. In 2000, the CMO had recommended that research on animal-human hybrid embryos should be banned. At first the government agreed, publishing a White Paper in 2006 which proposed a ban, while giving Parliament powers to create exceptions if more evidence about the potential of this research emerged in the future. John Gillott has suggested that this initial scepticism had its roots in the Bovine Spongiform Encephalopathy (BSE) crisis, which had crippled British farming and led to intense concern about the human variation of BSE, variant Creutzfeldt-Jacob Disease, as well as to wider anxiety about the governance of science. Just a year later, however, the government changed its mind, following the House of Commons Select Committee on Science and Technology's conclusion that hybrid research was necessary and should be permitted, provided that these embryos were also subject to the 14 day limit.

There are many different ways of combining human and animal DNA in order to create hybrid embryos. At the start of the twenty-first century, the hybrid embryos that scientists were most interested in creating would be created through CNR, using denucleated animal eggs and human nuclear DNA. These embryos would contain only mitochondrial animal DNA (the DNA in the outer 'shell' of the denucleated egg). At the time, it was believed that they would contain mainly human DNA, and that any stem cell lines extracted from them would be 100 per cent human.

Following an intensive public consultation exercise, the HFEA decided in September 2007 that licensing the creation of this sort of hybrid embryo lay within its statutory powers under the original legislation. Relying upon the House of Lords judgment in Quintavalle, the HFEA concluded that these embryos are within the same 'genus of fact' as other embryos covered by the 1990 Act: that is, they have a full human nuclear genome and are live.

The HFEA also took into account that Parliament's intention was for the regulatory scheme to be comprehensive, and 'there was to be no free for all'. If these human admixed embryos were not covered by the 1990 Act, then there would be no restrictions upon their creation. Because the intention was to retrieve animal eggs from abattoirs, their use would not be subject to the rules which govern research on animals, administered by the Home Office. If neither the Home Office nor the HFEA had any powers to control the creation and use of hybrid embryos, scientists could mix animal and human material in their garden sheds, keep them indefinitely, and do whatever they like to them.

In deciding that the creation of hybrid embryos could be licensed under the Act, the HFEA's press release made it clear that 'in making its decision it has not given a 'total green light' to cytoplasmic hybrids but only that such procedures can 'with caution and careful scrutiny, be permitted''. The strictness of the rules, including the 14 day limit, thus enabled the HFEA to make a liberalising decision, while simultaneously stressing that it was not opening the floodgates to anything.

The HFEA's Research Licence Committee issued the first two licences for research projects which intended to use animal eggs to create admixed embryos in January 2008, and a third was licensed a few months later. Scientists announced in April 2008 that they had successfully created the first animal/human hybrid embryo.

Predictably, the decision to grant these first licences to carry out research using animal eggs was challenged in the courts. Comment on Reproductive Ethics (CORE) and the Christian Legal Centre sought judicial review of the Research Licence Committee's decision, on the grounds that the HFEA had acted outside of its powers because these embryos are not 'human', and are therefore not regulated by the 1990 Act.

Before the case came to court, Parliament had enacted the 2008 amendments to the 1990 Act, although they were not yet in force. The creation of admixed embryos was one of the most controversial provisions in the amending legislation, and MPs had been given a free vote on the issue. A minority of parliamentarians were strongly opposed to the creation of human admixed embryos, and resistant to the idea that regulation was a panacea. Edward Leigh MP, for example, said:

> Do we want to put all our faith in regulation? Can we not recognise a principle when we see it? We do not have to be Christians to believe that we are all created in God's image. We can surely accept that embryos contain the genetic make-up of a complete human being and that we cannot and should not be spliced together with the animal kingdom.
>
> (HC Deb 19 May 2008)

More commonly, regulation was regarded more positively. Given the strictness of the rules to which human embryo research was subjected, John Bercow MP asked why an admixed embryo should be given even more protection:

> Why does he think that the admixed embryo – given that there will be licence conditions, and given the 14-day destruction rule – should have greater legal protection than the human embryo? So far, that point remains blindingly unclear.
>
> (HC Deb 19 May 2008)

The amending statute was passed, and the changes it made to the 1990 Act mean that the Act now specifically permits the creation of human admixed embryos for research purposes, subject to all of the other restrictions on embryo research, such as the 14 day limit.

The fact that Parliament had expressed its intention to permit the creation of human admixed embryos made it difficult for CORE and the Christian Legal Centre to argue that granting licences for this sort of research was contrary to the intention of Parliament. In December 2008, in *R (on the application of Quintavalle and CLC) v HFEA* (2008), Dobbs J refused to grant permission for leave to apply for judicial review of the HFEA's decision to grant the first two licences, describing the application as 'entirely without merit'.

The 1990 Act did not define the word 'human', and Dobbs LJ thought that the HFEA's legal advice – namely that it should take a cautious approach and treat such embryos as human to ensure that they are regulated – was in accordance with the spirit and purpose of the 1990 Act. She also noted that Parliament had made its intention in relation to hybrid embryos clear, and that the scientists who had received the first two licences to carry out this research would, even if the original Licence Committee decision was struck down, be able to reapply for their licences when the new Act came into force in October 2009.

The Liberalising Impact of Strict Boundaries

One of the key points in this chapter is that the set of strict regulatory boundaries contained in the original 1990 Act, of which the 14 day limit is the paradigmatic example, has in practice enabled future expansion of the rules. This is important for several reasons, including the basic Warnockian point that since laws are expressive of social values, it is not surprising that they change – and nor should it be. To Warnock, it was the role of the law as a formal instrument of moral expression that mattered most: to have a law regulating sensitive matters such as human embryo research was morally preferable to not having one. But this is an argument about moral principle being manifest as form, not content. Logically, the formal function of having a law rather than not having one is unchanged if the content of that law is amended. Repeatedly, people advocating for extensions to the 14 day rule, both inside and outside Parliament, have therefore accurately cited the robustness of regulation as a compelling reason why it is entirely possible to view the historic process of gradual extensions to the definition of permissible research as proof that the foundational legislative principles are reaffirmed rather than diminished by serial amendments. In other words, bright clear lines are essential – but this does not mean they cannot be changed, or that different lines would not be equally effective.

It is precisely the robustness of the legal framework governing human fertilisation and embryology in the UK, moreover, and its ability to be successfully adapted over time (indeed repeatedly, and over quite a long period of time), that has put paid to the slippery slope fears about the 'door being opened' to new entities and techniques such as hESCs, human admixed embryos and therapeutic cloning. Indeed all of these unanticipated developments have been swiftly, firmly and straightforwardly dealt with through new statutory provisions – even when they concern scientific developments considered biologically impossible at the time the initial legislation was drafted, or topics about which the public have unusually strong feelings, such as cloning. There is ample evidence too that amendments such as these have increased public trust in the ability of government to devise appropriate and balanced, as well as robust and effective, legislation to address controversial subjects such as human cloning.

This is not to say that public concerns about human embryo research and new areas such as embryo modelling should not continue to be the subject of robust public, professional and parliamentary consultation and debate, however. Among other things, such debates are essential to keep track of the issues that concern people and why – especially in relation to complex subjects such as gene editing, artificial gametes, and embryo models. It is also important, both sociologically and for governance purposes, to keep track of how the legacy of the UK's legislation, and the accompanying expansion of both research and treatment this has enabled, have influenced the public's views of experiments involving human embryos. After all, this has been an area of immense social, technological and scientific change over the past half-century. When embryo research was debated in the 1980s, IVF had not yet touched many people's lives, whereas today almost everyone knows someone who has been affected by IVF. Although it remains unclear how much therapeutic benefit hES or iPS cells can bring, and many other regenerative medical possibilities remain at an early stage, there is no doubt that IVF has had significant translational success. The rapid expansion of IVF technology, moreover, has so normalised and naturalised the test-tube baby that this term itself evokes a different era. Sociologically, we might consider the 'IVF effect' to have had a generally positive effect on public perceptions of the benefits that can be gained from basic scientific research. There is some evidence as well that both the Warnock Consensus and the IVF effect have significantly softened public perceptions of the possibility of using new techniques such as gene editing for reproductive purposes (Kaur 2022). In 2023 when the news broke that new embryo models created without the use of egg or sperm were capable of high levels of autonomous self-organisation and 'complete' development, we did not see the dozens of 'Franken' headlines that often used to accompany such announcements. Indeed, even the simultaneous news that such models existed in the same 'legal vacuum' as that into which Louise Brown was born appeared to cause relatively little controversy. To the contrary, such developments clearly appear to garner much greater public support than in the past, and although there is no definitive evidence to prove that the rapid normalisation of IVF has played a significant causal role in this shift in public perceptions of reproductive science and biomedicine, we can nonetheless speculate that this is highly likely to be the case. For example, when the Human Developmental Biology Initiative (HDBI) carried out public dialogue workshops with 70 members of the public in the summer of 2023, more or less concurrent with the news announcing the embryo modelling breakthroughs, they found that 'improvement to IVF [was] one of the clearest areas in which participants place their hopes for research with early human embryos' (HDBI 2023). Aside from those who have 'in principle' objections to any type of embryo research, as well as IVF, based on religious scripture, most of the HDBI consultation participants were more concerned with the suffering caused by IVF's low success rates, inadequate NHS funding for infertility treatment, and the need for better fertility care in general than embryo protection.

In contrast to the slippery slope fears that appear to have been largely contradicted by the speed and firmly principled handling of numerous controversial scientific innovations over the last four decades, it appears that human fertilisation and embryology is an area in which public trust has been strengthened, due in no small part to an active, ongoing and genuine dialogue between members of the public, the relevant professional bodies, government, academia, regulators and many other organisations from the third sector such as charities, think tanks and patient groups. The existence of a tried-and-tested regulatory regime, coupled with greater public familiarity with IVF – and importantly also IVF failure – has helped to foster a climate in which there is considerable sympathy for the goals of embryo research. This improved climate for translational reproductive biomedicine does not imply that the public are now unconcerned about the manipulation of human embryos, or in particular the possible use of such embryos for reproductive purposes. Indeed it is especially vital to continue to research public attitudes and views toward the use of human embryos for research purposes precisely because we should assume such attitudes and views are complex and multifaceted, as well as diverse, emotive and often strongly held.

Notes

1 First reported in Handyside et al. (1990). Five days before a House of Commons vote on the Human Fertilisation and Embryology Bill, newspapers published a picture of Professor Robert Winston with the pregnant women who would be the first to benefit from the new technique of preimplantation genetic testing when their healthy children were born in a few months' time (Mulkay 1997).
2 As the feminist political scientist Rosalind Petchesky first pointed out in the 1980s, Pro-Life leaders have 'made a conscious strategic shift from religious discourses and authorities to medico-technical ones in [their] efforts to win over the courts, the legislatures and popular "hearts and minds"' (1987: 58). This strategy is also evident in the use of graphic imagery of aborted fetuses as a religious campaigning strategy.
3 Of course, opposition to 'destructive embryo research' still exists. See, for example, Wills (2001) and Jones (2011).
4 In fact many fewer eggs, donated by Hwang's research assistants, were used, and the data fabricated. Hwang was subsequently convicted and imprisoned for his crimes.

References

Baylis, Françoise (2009) 'The HFEA public consultation process on hybrids and chimeras: informed, effective, and meaningful?' *Kennedy Institute of Ethics Journal* 19(1): 41–62.
Deech, Ruth (2002) 'Regulation of therapeutic cloning in the UK' *Reproductive BioMedicine Online* 5(1): 7–11.
Gillott, John (2013) 'The changing governance of embryo research?' (2013) *New Genetics and Society* 32(2): 190–206.

Golombok, Susan (2020) *We are family: The modern transformation of parents and children* (Scribe).

Handyside, Alan H., Kontogianni, Elena H., Hardy, K.R.M.L. and Winston, Robert M.L. (1990) 'Pregnancies from biopsied human preimplantation embryos sexed by Y-specific DNA amplification' (1990) *Nature* 344: 768–770.

HDBI (2023) *Public dialogue on research involving early human embryos* (Human Developmental Biology Initiative).

Herrmann, Svea Luise (2003) 'Deregulation via regulation: on the moralisation and naturalisation of embryonic stem cell research in the British parliamentary debates of 2000/2001' *Österreichische Zeitschrift für Politikwissenschaft* 32(2): 149–161.

HFEA (2004) *Thirteenth annual report* (Human Fertilisation and Embryology Authority).

House of Commons (2004) *Human reproductive technologies and the law: fifth report of session 2004–05* (House of Commons Science and Technology Committee).

House of Commons (2007) *Government proposals for the regulation of hybrid and chimera embryos: fifth report of session 2006–7* (House of Commons Science and Technology Committee).

House of Lords (2002) *Stem cell research* (House of Lords Select Committee on Stem Cell Research).

Jones, David (2011) 'The "special status" of the human embryo in the United Kingdom: an exploration of the use of language in public policy' *Human Reproduction & Genetic Ethics* 17: 66–83.

Lovell-Badge, Robin (2008) 'The regulation of human embryo and stem-cell research in the United Kingdom' *Nature Reviews Molecular Cell Biology* 9(12): 998–1003.

Mulkay, Michael (1997) *The embryo research debate: science and the politics of reproduction* (Cambridge University Press).

O'Neill, Onora (2003) 'Stem cells: ethics, legislation and regulation' *Comptes Rendus Biologies* 326(7): 673–676.

Petchesky, Rosalind (1987) 'The power of visual culture in the politics of reproduction' *Feminist Studies* 13(2): 263–292.

Plomer, Aurora (2002) 'Beyond the HFE Act 1990: the regulation of stem cell research in the UK' *Medical Law Review* 10(2): 132.

Progress Educational Trust (2022) *Fertility, genomics and embryo research: public attitudes and understanding* (PET).

Stojkovic, Miodrag et al. (2005) 'Derivation of a human blastocyst after heterologous nuclear transfer to donated oocytes' *Reproductive Biomedicine Online* 11(2): 226–231.

Thomson, J.A. et al. (1998) 'Embryonic stem cell lines derived from human blastocysts' *Science* 282(5391): 1145–1147.

Wills, Susan E. (2001) 'Federal funding of human embryonic stem cell research: illegal, unethical and unnecessary' *Journal of Contemporary Health Law & Policy* 18: 95.

Wilmut, Ian, Schnieke, Angelika E., McWhir, Jim, Kind, Alexander J. and Campbell, Keith H.S. (1997) 'Viable offspring derived from fetal and adult mammalian cells' *Nature* 385: 810–813.

Legal Judgments

R (on the application of Quintavalle) v Secretary of State for Health [2003] UKHL 13.

R (on the application of Quintavalle and CLC) v HFEA (2008) [2008] EWHC 3395 (Admin).

Parliamentary Debates

HC Deb (23 November 1984) vol. 68 col. 565.
HC Deb (4 February 1988) vol. 126 cols 1200, 1210, 1221, 1222.
HC Deb (23 April 1990) vol. 171 cols 57, 84, 90.
HC Deb (15 December 2000) vol. 359 cols 894–895, 902.
HC Deb (19 December 2000) vol. 360 cols 215, 218.
HL Deb (22 January 2001) vol. 621 cols 21–22, 24, 53.
HC Deb (29 November 2001) vol. 375 col. 1200.
HC Deb (19 May 2008) vol. 476 cols 28, 44, 63.
HL Deb (31 October 1984) vol. 456 col. 564.
HL Deb (15 January 1988) vol. 491 col. 1504.
HL Deb (7 December 1989) vol. 513 col. 1057.
HL Deb (4 February 1990) vol. 515 cols 969, 979.

6 The Future of the 14 Day Rule

In this chapter, we turn from considering the lessons learned from its origins and history to explore the future of the 14 day limit. As we have seen, two scientific developments, in particular, raise questions about the continued viability of an absolute bar on embryo research after 14 days. First, reports that scientists had been able to keep embryos alive *in vitro* for 13 days (before they were destroyed in order not to breach the 14 day limit) have led some to argue that the limit should be increased (Hyun et al. 2016; Harris 2016). Extending the limit would allow us to find out more about embryo development, especially during the critical (but until now inaccessible) window of 14–28 days (Hyun et al. 2021), when embryo research is prohibited and it is impossible to carry out research using miscarried or aborted embryos (McCully 2021). Secondly, the creation of embryo-like models raises the question of how they should be treated morally as well as legally, in terms of governance and regulation. How 'like' an embryo do entities, cells and materials have to be in order to be treated as if they *were* an embryo? This question is clearly important to the public, and to government, but it is also essential for the scientific community, and especially for scientific teams working with human embryo models, who need clear guidelines as to what is permissible or not.

Before addressing the question of whether the limit should remain as it is or be extended, and whether or how any time limit ought to apply to embryo models, it is important to be clear about why the 14 day limit matters. What functions, exactly, is it fulfilling? Is it simply important that there is a clear, bright-line rule, but where the line is drawn can, like other rules, be changed, so that 21 or 28 days could serve the same purpose of providing a clear and readily understandable, albeit less restrictive limit on research? Alternatively, is it the 'biological' explanation for the 14 day rule (the emergence of the primitive streak and the fact that twinning is no longer possible) which is critical, in which case extending the limit would be feasible only if a new 'objective' biological marker could be identified, which could be used to justify extending the legal time limit beyond 14 days?

Although our starting point is the 14 day limit in UK law, derived from the 1984 Warnock Report, we noted earlier that it is 'one of the most internationally agreed rules in reproductive science and medicine to date' (Appleby and Bredenoord 2018). As we have seen, it applies in at least 12 countries worldwide (Matthews

DOI: 10.4324/9781003294108-6

and Moralí 2020), and in jurisdictions which permit embryo research with no time limit, 'scientists have voluntarily complied with this limitation' (Suter 2022).

Of course, there are countries where all embryo research is illegal,[1] but the degree of international consensus around the 14 day limit is remarkable. It is normal for different jurisdictions to exercise a wide 'margin of appreciation' when regulating matters which touch on the moral status of the embryo/fetus (O'Donovan 2006). Within the European Union (EU), for example, despite progressive harmonisation of rules concerning trade, employment and consumer protection, there is no consensus on the regulation of abortion, surrogacy and fertility treatment, and laws vary widely across the EU. Harmonisation of abortion law between the US and the UK is unimaginable. In almost all respects, there is huge variety worldwide in the regulation of the treatment of embryos/fetuses, which makes the 14 day rule stand out as a rare example of widespread (if not universal) international consensus.

There may be considerable value in trying to retain this international consensus (Williams and Johnson 2020), whether that means leaving the limit at 14 days, or seeking international agreement for a new time limit. If only one country extended its limit, it might be likely to become an attractive destination for scientists who are unable to carry out research after 14 days in their own countries. Peng et al. (2022) also note that researchers from the first jurisdiction to extend the limit will be able to maximise future profits by 'developing [a] global patent portfolio'. With a worldwide consensus on the time limit for embryo research, countries are not in competition with each other for scientific expertise and funding, and cross-national research collaboration is facilitated.

In May 2021, the International Society for Stem Cell Research (ISSCR) published revised guidelines, which for the first time indicated that it might be legitimate to carry out research after 14 days. Interestingly, however, the ISSCR did not recommend a new time limit, or a new developmental landmark to replace the primitive streak (Sawai et al. 2021). The ISSCR (2021) instead agreed to remove 'culture of human embryos beyond 14 days or primitive streak formation' from the category of 'prohibited activities', and called for:

> national academies of science, academic societies, funders, and regulators to lead public conversations touching on the scientific significance as well as the societal and ethical issues raised by allowing such research. Should broad public support be achieved within a jurisdiction, and if local policies and regulations permit, a specialized scientific and ethical oversight process could weigh whether the scientific objectives necessitate and justify the time in culture beyond 14 days, ensuring that only a minimal number of embryos are used to achieve the research objectives.

ISSCR guidelines are re-evaluated every five years, which means that now is 'the time for the community to engage in meaningful and substantial public communication and deliberations' (Clark et al. 2021). The ISSCR is therefore advocating public engagement on whether the 14 day rule should be extended, rather than its immediate replacement with a more permissive limit. Nevertheless, there has been criticism of the ISSCR for not recommending a new time limit, while at the same time suggesting that 14 days could legitimately be exceeded (Johnston et al. 2021), and for advocating public engagement, while not having consulted the public before revising its own guidelines (Subbaraman 2021).

In Limits We Trust?

Jonathan Montgomery (2017) has explained that the 14 day limit 'distinguishes ethical questions that are to be regarded as closed from those which are to be treated as open to further reflection'. Beyond 14 days, 'the law has determined that the moral value of the embryo will always preclude the pursuit of knowledge through research', regardless of the value of the knowledge that could be generated as a result. In contrast, before 14 days, the HFEA must undertake a 'balancing exercise' in order to determine whether the statutory criteria for a licence have been satisfied in the individual case. There is therefore no *carte blanche* for scientists before 14 days, rather it is only in the window between fertilisation and 14 days that it is possible to mount a claim that research on embryos could be justifiable.

As we have seen, the 14 day limit's complexity comes from the fact that it is many different things at the same time. First, on the one hand, it is an essentially arbitrary regulatory limit: an embryo at 15 days is not very different from an embryo at 14 days, but a line needs to be drawn somewhere, and drawing it at 14 days appears to be reasonable and publicly acceptable, as well as providing a clear and unambiguous boundary between lawful and unlawful practices. As Mary Warnock (2017) explained, if the limitation were expressed only in terms of the embryo's stage of development, a scientist might be able to claim 'that this embryo was developing in an exceptional way or unusually slowly'. Such claims would have to be investigated on a case-by-case basis, which would itself be expensive and time-consuming. In contrast, as Warnock (2017) put it, 'everyone can count up to 14, and everyone can keep and examine records'.

An analogy could be drawn with other statutory time limits, such as the age at which someone is allowed to drive and vote. In the UK, we do not allow a teenager to drive and vote only when she can prove that she is able to control a car and exercise political judgement. Instead, it is sensible to have a universal minimum age for driving and voting, and in the UK, 17 and 18 have been chosen as reasonable limits (and other countries have made different choices), even though we know that a child does not instantaneously acquire the ability to drive safely on their 17th birthday, or the capacity to make political choices precisely a year later.

On the other hand, 14 days is not arbitrary 'in the sense of being random and without reasoned basis' (Montgomery 2017). As we have seen, the Warnock Committee did not pluck 14 days out of thin air, and there is a biological justification for choosing 14 days: this is when the first signs of the primitive streak appear, and after which twinning is no longer possible. As Mary Warnock explained in a television interview, 'before fourteen days the embryo hasn't decided how many people it is going to be' (quoted in Lockwood 1988).

The appearance of the primitive streak indicates 'that the embryo proper is beginning differentiation and development as an organised individual' (NIH Ad Hoc Group of Consultants to the Advisory Committee to the Director 1994), and represents 'the first point in embryonic development at which it could be said that a potential human being exists' (Elves and McGuinness 2017). It is also around the time that an in vivo embryo implants in the pregnant woman's uterus, and after which the central nervous system begins to develop. As Anne McLaren (1984) said of it: 'If I had to point to a stage and say "This is when I began being me", I would think it would have to be here.' In the US, the controversial Catholic theologian Charles Curran, who was quoted in the first public document to recommend that there should be a 14 day limit to the growth of the human embryo *in vitro* (a 1979 report of the Ethics Advisory Board of the US Department of Health, Education and Welfare), argued that a human being cannot exist before 14 days gestation, and that 'human life is not present until individuality is established' (Curran 1973; Diamond 1975).

The limit is therefore both a number of days (for clarity's sake) and a significant biological marker (which demonstrates why this is a reasonable place to draw the line). It is, therefore, simultaneously arbitrary and justifiable. As Mary Warnock (2017) has explained: 'The number 14 was *not* arbitrary in the sense that we drew it out of a hat. But it *was* arbitrary in the sense that it might have been a different number, though not very greatly different.'

An analogy could be drawn with abortion. As early as 1115, 'quickening', or when the woman could first feel the fetus move inside her, was a biological milestone which was invoked in order to distinguish between abortion as a misdemeanour and as a more serious crime, akin to homicide. Now, it is common for abortion laws to rely upon fetal viability as a rough proxy for the point beyond which abortion is lawful only in exceptional circumstances, for example, to save the woman's life or because the fetus has a grave congenital anomaly. In order for the law to be able to draw clear lines, the limit tends to be expressed in numerical terms, as 24 weeks in the case of the UK, or until the overturning of *Roe v Wade* (1973) in the US,[2] the end of the second trimester.

Reliance on the potential for individuation as the point beyond which research is unlawful is itself interesting, because being used in a research project will preclude an individual embryo from becoming a person, so its potential for individuation is in practice purely theoretical (Appleby and Bredenoord 2018). Some embryos that are donated to research are so chromosomally or morphologically abnormal that they could never result in a pregnancy, let alone the birth of a child, but the regulation of embryo research does not distinguish between those embryos that do and those that do not have the potential to become a person. Rather all embryos, including those with no actual potential at all, are covered by regulation. It is therefore not that the potential for individuation is present in the *individual embryo* which is used in a research project; rather, potential exists in the abstract, for embryos *as a class*, even though it is 'only in utero embryos [that] have "active potential"' (Sawai et al. 2020).

Even if we are concerned with the properties of embryos in the abstract, it is also worth noting that monozygotic twinning is very unusual (occurring in 3 or 4 in 1000 births), so that 'an individual is almost always present much earlier than 14 days' (Blackshaw and Rodger 2021). Michael Lockwood (1988) has pointed out a further paradox in relying on 'potential' to ground the 14 day limit. Keeping an embryo *in vitro* for longer periods of time does not increase the embryo's potential. On the contrary:

> if we're talking about embryos outside the womb, it isn't true, even as a rule, that the older it is the greater is the likelihood that, were it to be transferred to a womb, it would develop into a human person. For beyond a certain stage, the likelihood that it could be successfully implanted will begin to decline sharply: the time will come when it will, so to speak, have missed the boat.

Even more unusual is the possibility of the converse of twinning, where two embryos fuse to become a single embryo, so that what was two potential individuals becomes one.

Secondly, we have suggested that the 14 day limit represents a compromise in circumstances where consensus is impossible, but it could also be argued that there is no compromise involved at all. On the one hand, those who object to embryo research in principle and those who are in favour of a longer time limit are never going to agree with each other. At one end of the spectrum, some people believe that research on embryos is never justifiable, while at the other, it might be argued that research should be possible on embryos whenever scientists might be able to derive useful information. As with abortion, a compromise is devised, using time limits and other restrictions, so that abortion and embryo research are lawful in certain circumstances, but are not permissible at any gestational stage 'on demand'.

In relation to embryo research, the 14 day limit is a compromise which permits embryo research, but only within a strict time limit, and subject to other restrictions – including that the use of embryos is necessary, and that the research is carried out only for tightly specified purposes – which make it clear that there is to be no 'free for all' (*R (on the application of Quintavalle) v Secretary of State for Health* 2003, *per* Lord Bingham at [13]). The 14 day limit on embryo research responds to those who raise the 'slippery slope' concern that experimenting on embryos is the first step to experimenting on sentient beings by absolutely prohibiting research long before sentience is achieved. As Josephine Johnston put it, 'It was a political decision to show the public there is a framework for this research, that we aren't growing babies in labs' (quoted in Regaldo 2021).

On the other hand, because in 1990 and for 26 years afterwards, it was not possible to keep an intact embryo alive *in vitro* for more than about 7 days,[3] this could be said to be a rather peculiar 'compromise'. Elves and McGuinness (2017) point out that the *Oxford English Dictionary* defines compromise as 'an intermediate state between conflicting opinions, reached by mutual concession'. In 1990, 14 days did not involve any practical concession from scientists, rather 14 days allowed research for as long as it was scientifically possible, and 'gave scientists virtually everything they needed at the time' (Devolder 2017). Only since 2016 has 14 days represented a compromise between those who want to carry out research for longer than this, and those who believe either that that would be a step too far, or that all embryo research is fundamentally immoral.

As Katrien Devolder points out, the fact that when the 14 day limit was set, this was around twice as long as it was technically possible to culture an intact embryo *in vitro* 'may create the impression that the 14-day limit was adopted to gain the acceptance of the public and policymakers so that scientists could proceed with their scientific research'. As we have seen, Mary Warnock did not see regulation as an impediment to medical and scientific progress. Rather, as Duncan Wilson (2011) has explained, the system of regulation was intended to *protect* doctors and scientists, allowing scientists 'to get on with their work, without the fear of private prosecutions, or disruption by those who object to what they are doing' (Warnock 1985a). In short, the best way to deflect calls for new technologies to be banned was to demonstrate that they could instead by controlled and contained within what looked like strict limits, set down in legislation.

As we have frequently noted throughout this book, the logics of 14 day limit are recombinant: they amalgamate a pragmatic political solution based on regulatory proposals with a basis in both common sense and textbook biology to resolve a fundamental moral question (Elves and McGuinness 2017). Biological facts – the appearance of the primitive streak and the individuation of the embryo – provide a basis for a time limit to address the problem of when it could be legitimate to experiment upon the earliest form of human life from the logistical and strategic point of view of how not to end up failing in that task. Meeting all of these objectives at once with any one of these forms of reasoning was unlikely to have succeeded without the others.

On the one hand, many would accept that 14 days does not represent a definitive conclusion about when an embryo acquires moral status. Supporters of the 14 day limit do not generally believe that an embryo acquires moral status at 14 days (Hyun et al. 2021), or that 14 days represents the definitive dividing line between ethical and unethical research. A much more common view remains the one advocated by Warnock herself, and now enshrined in UK law, where it has been repeatedly reaffirmed, namely that it is important to have a limit, and that 14 days is a reasonable place to draw the line. On this view, the 14 day limit does not embody a view about what an embryo's moral status is, and when it acquires it. Rather, it is a political and pragmatic solution to the problem of fundamental moral disagreement. To some, this is explicitly a logic of compromise. To others, such as Warnock, it was a morally responsible solution to the sociological fact that no single position on the wide spectrum of opinion about human embryo research could legitimately be deemed absolutely right or wrong.

Indeed, in her 2004 memoir, *Nature and Morality,* Mary Warnock describes the exact point in the Committee's deliberations when she realised that instead of talking about what was morally right or wrong, the Committee instead needed to focus upon what was *acceptable* (Warnock 2004). Their task was not to determine whether embryo research could be morally justifiable, but to come up with recommendations that would be acceptable to Parliament and the general public. Indeed, as Mary Warnock said herself in the introduction to her original Report, she 'would not dispute' the judgement of others that that her Committee's Report was 'short on imagination and long on pragmatism' (Warnock 1985b).

Yet, on the other hand, defining the embryo before 14 days as a 'pre-embryo', in order to distinguish it from the 'embryo proper', which exists only after 14 days, might facilitate treating them as different entities. For example, Anne McLaren (1990) argued that before *individual* embryonic development began – that is, before 14 days – the term conceptus or pre-embryo was more appropriate. For a few years in the 1980s, the word pre-embryo, with its implication that there is something special and different about very early human embryos (Jasanoff 2011), was in common usage. Colomer and Pastor (2012) have pointed out that once embryo research had become lawful and widely accepted, the term pre-embryo largely disappeared. By then, they argue, it had served its purpose.

It is, however, noteworthy that the *Oxford English Dictionary*'s definition of embryo (as 'the unborn human offspring, especially during the early stages of development'), is further fleshed out as follows:

> The term is now most narrowly applied to the human organism from the point, *usually in the second week after fertilization and just prior to implantation,* when its cells become differentiated from those of the trophoblast, until the end of the eighth week, when the organs begin to develop and it is termed a *fetus* [our emphasis].

While most scientists would use the term 'embryo' before the second week after fertilisation, there are still those who believe that there is something fundamentally different about embryos before and after around 14 days. Ted Peters (2021), for example, sets out the morally relevant changes that occur between 12 and 14 days, and claims not only that 'there is no point beyond 14 days when such a relevant collection of events occurs', but also that this cluster of events indicates that 'nature is trying to communicate to our conscience'.

Fourthly, the 14 day limit is part of a cluster of restrictions which are intended to indicate that the early human embryo is 'special' and should be treated with 'respect' (Warnock Committee 1984). Yet at the same time, the 14 day limit facilitates the instrumental use and destruction of early human embryos, which we would ordinarily consider a peculiar way to show respect. Dan Callahan (1995) describes this as an 'odd form of esteem – at once high-minded and altogether lethal. What in the world can that kind of respect mean?' As Catriona McMillan (2021) has pointed out, it is 'difficult to enable a "middle position" between protection and destruction in practice; we either allow embryos to be destroyed, or we do not'. If the 'special' status of the embryo does not require us to act in a particular way towards it, is it merely a rhetorical device (Ford 2009), or a 'legal and ethical comfort blanket' (McMillan 2021)?

Alternatively, as Michael Sandel has explained, it may be 'a mistake to claim respect is all or nothing, on or off' (quoted in Steinbock 2007). Instead, Steinbock (2007) suggests that it may it possible to show respect for embryos not only 'by treating them as inviolable and prohibiting embryo research', but also 'by placing restrictions on their use':

> Respect for embryos rules out frivolous or trivial uses, such as using human embryos to create jewelry or cosmetics. These are situations in which there

is no need to use human embryos and their use displays contempt rather than respect for human life. However, respect for human life does not rule out significant research that could cure devastating diseases or save lives – indeed, quite the contrary.[4]

Mary Warnock has subsequently acknowledged that it might have been better not to use the word respect, and that *non-frivolity* better captures what the Committee meant:

> I regret that in the original report that led up to the 1990 legislation we used words such as 'respect for the embryo'. That seems to me to lead to certain absurdities. You cannot respectfully pour something down the sink – which is the fate of the embryo after it has been used for research, or if it is not going to be used for research or for anything else. I think that what we meant by the rather foolish expression 'respect' was that the early embryo should never be used frivolously for research purposes.
>
> (HL Deb 5 December 2002)

Finally, there both is and is not a close analogy between research on embryos and research on animals. On the one hand, and especially in the case of research on non-human primates, both research on embryos and research on animals could be said to involve experimenting on entities with intermediate moral status – neither the full status of a human being, nor that of an inanimate object. The embryo is not a person, but it is also 'not nothing' (*St George's Healthcare NHS Trust v S* (1998)). Animals too are not things, but rather are sentient beings, whose instrumental use requires justification. Mary Warnock has said that in both cases,

> the essential instrument of regulation is a body, either statutory or set up by an Act of Parliament, which has overall responsibility for the control demanded but is independent of government and is composed not solely of experts or specialists but to a great extent of lay members of the public who are interested, in the sense of being concerned, but who have no commercial or scientific axe to grind.
>
> (Warnock 1985b)

In the case of both animals and embryos, licences can be issued only to people who are able to persuade the licensing body that the research would (a) be valuable, and (b) could not be carried out without using animals or embryos. In both cases, it is possible to revoke licences, and there are criminal offences to back up the licensing regime.

In addition, it has been suggested that the 3Rs (replacement, reduction and refinement) approach to the ethics of animal experimentation could be adapted for research on embryos (Moris et al. 2021). This might, for example, lead to a presumption that scientists should not carry out research on embryos when the research could be done on stem cell-based embryo models.

On the other hand, there are important differences between the regulation of animal research and research on embryos; in particular, there is no time limit for animal research: research either is permissible or is not. The licensing body must decide that the research can take place, or refuse a licence. There is no scope for allowing research, but only within a brief window of time. More fundamentally, it could be argued that the 3Rs approach is a poor fit for embryo research, because embryos which are not going to be used in treatment would otherwise be discarded, and it is hard to see how throwing away a potentially valuable scientific resource is morally preferable to learning something from it.

The Future of the 14 Day Limit: Justifying an Extension beyond 14 Days

As we have seen, after about 28 days, it is possible to carry out research on embryos that have been miscarried or aborted. It is therefore the 14–28 day period which is currently a 'black box', when research cannot be carried out even though we know that significant changes are happening to the embryo. The emergence of the primitive streak marks the start of gastrulation, 'a process whereby the embryonic inner cell mass starts to differentiate into three layers (endoderm, mesoderm, and ectoderm)' (Cavaliere 2017). In weeks three and four, the developmental events 'are entirely distinct from the processes of blastula formation and implantation in weeks one and two, and therefore are of unique interest for understanding the genetic and environmental basis of birth defects' (Chen and Chisholm 2017).

In order to extend the 14 day limit, it is widely accepted that several prerequisites would have to be met. First, a persuasive case would have to be made that an extension would be likely to lead to scientific gains, which in turn are likely to have a demonstrably positive impact on patients. For example, carrying out research between 14–28 days might enable us to better understand and hence prevent unexplained early pregnancy loss. The majority of IVF embryos fail to implant. Around 25 per cent of 'natural' pregnancies fail in the first seven weeks, 'largely due to defects in development' (Zernicka-Goetz 2017). In addition, 'many new-borns die within weeks of birth every year due to congenital anomalies (mainly abnormalities in heart and neural tube development)', and the 14–28 day period is a crucial stage in the development of the heart and neural tube. It might therefore be possible to establish that an extension to the 14 day limit could improve people's lives, by reducing the frequency of pregnancy loss, increasing IVF success rates, and reducing the number of babies born with potentially fatal congenital anomalies. In addition, research during this period might be able to establish whether chromosomal anomalies identified using PGT-A (preimplantation genetic testing for aneuploidy) are 'true anomalies' or whether, as some research appears to indicate, they will sometimes resolve themselves (Suter 2021).

Two other reasons for extending the limit are, first, in order to validate stem-cell based embryo-models, discussed below, and, secondly, enabling more comprehensive evaluation of the safety and efficacy of current and future innovations in fertility treatment, such as mitochondrial replacement, *in vitro* gametogenesis (IVG) and human genome editing (Lovell-Badge et al. 2021). If, for example, it becomes possible to eliminate the need for gamete donation, by enabling people who do not have functioning gametes to make egg and sperm from induced pluripotent stem cells, it will be necessary to establish that if these IVG gametes are used in fertility treatment, the resulting embryos are likely to develop normally after cell differentiation begins.

Of course, one obvious difficulty with establishing that valuable research could take place after 14 days is that it is difficult to *prove* that it would, because at the moment, culturing embryos for longer than 14 days is unlawful. Indeed, at the time of writing, we do not know whether it is possible to culture an embryo for longer than 14 days, because the researchers who came close to this limit in 2016 were under a duty to dispose of the embryos at 13 days. Nevertheless, evidence that macaque embryos have been cultured for about 20 days, which is significantly beyond the equivalent of the 14 day limit in human embryos, suggests that extending the limit could be feasible (Ma et al. 2019).

Secondly, it would be necessary to establish that this valuable research would not be possible *unless* the time limit for embryo research were extended beyond 14 days (Devolder 2017). Because scientists' ability to culture embryos *in vitro* between 7–14 days is relatively new, 'the second week of embryonic development has only recently become accessible for study' (Clark et al. 2021). As a result, are we sure that making use of the research which is now possible on 7–14 day embryos could not provide the same benefits as are being claimed for research after 14 days? If 'there is still much to be learned between 7 and 14 days post fertilization' (Clark et al. 2021), opponents of an extension might argue that it would be premature. It would therefore be important for scientists to be able to explain why research on embryos after 14 days would be likely to yield valuable results that could not be obtained by adhering to the current 14 day limit.

Thirdly, it might be helpful to be able to explain what the benefits of embryo research thus far have been, so that it is clear that embryo research carried out under the existing time limit has delivered real, tangible benefits to patients, for example, by improving outcomes in IVF treatment. If there is doubt about whether the initial promise of embryo research has in fact been delivered, it will be harder to build support for extending its boundaries.

The Warnock Committee (1984) had been clear that if research on embryos were prohibited, 'IVF could not continue', because 'it would have been too risky for patients' (Warnock 2007), and a majority of the Committee did not regard the prohibition of IVF as 'a serious option'. In the 2020s, it seems unlikely that the UK Parliament would decide to ban IVF,[5] and it might therefore be important to explain once again that safe and effective IVF treatment would not possible without research on embryos.

In the US, 'embryo adoption' programmes commonly involve Pro-Life Christian couples who have undergone IVF, and as a result, have embryos left in storage, but who object to embryo destruction, and would not contemplate donation to research (Cromer 2023). This could be described as wilful blindness to the fact that embryo research is an essential precursor of IVF treatment. Evidence that continuous improvement in the safety and efficacy of IVF has been possible only thanks to embryo research will be helpful when making the claim that even more embryo research might be likely to lead to even better outcomes for patients.

Fourthly, if the 14 day limit were to change, it would have to be to a new time limit, which is clear, stable and robustly policed. As we have seen, the existence of a time limit is, in fact, helpful for scientists, by setting boundaries which allow them to 'get on with their work'. Most scientists are not arguing that the time limit should be lifted entirely. Calls are for a new time limit, not for no limit at all.

A further important feature of the 14 day limit proposed by the Warnock Committee is that it has 'teeth'. It is a criminal offence to culture an embryo for more than 14 days, and any scientist who did so could go to prison for up to 10 years (HFE Act 1990: section 41). Even if it could be argued that this penalty is unduly harsh (House of Commons 2004), retaining the criminal law as a buttress for the 14 day rule may be valuable in persuading people that a modest extension is not going to lead to 'a free for all'. This is important because one danger of extending the limit, even if only by a few days, is that, as Cavaliere explains, '"slippery slopers" might take this extension as a sign that their fears are well grounded' (Cavaliere 2017). It would therefore be important to ensure that any new limit remains fixed for a considerable period of time, and is enforced rigorously by the regulator.

Fifthly, it is taken for granted that, in the same way as the Warnock Report made recommendations that the Committee thought were likely to be acceptable as a matter of public policy, any change to the 14 day limit would have to be acceptable to the general public. A YouGov poll, carried out for the BBC in 2017 found that 48 per cent of the sample of 1740 respondents would be in favour of extending the limit, while 19 per cent were in favour of keeping the 14 day limit, 10 per cent would ban all embryo research, and 23 per cent did not express a view.[6] More recently, the Progress Educational Trust (2022) found more support for retaining the 14 day limit.

While opinion polls provide a useful snapshot of public opinion, it is important to acknowledge that many members of the public may not have a view about the time limit for embryo research, and indeed some may not know either that such a limit currently exists, or that embryo research is currently lawful. As a result, gauging the public acceptability of an increased time limit should involve public engagement, involvement and dialogue, as well as opinion polls and focus groups.

As we have seen, public engagement increasingly adopts 'what science communicators call a "dialogue model" rather than the "deficit model" of the past' (Hyun et al. 2021). The deficit model assumes 'the purpose of science communication is to "fill the knowledge gaps" in a largely one-way flow of information from expert to layperson' (Reincke et al. 2020). In contrast, the dialogue model involves a 'two-way flow of information from expert to layperson and vice versa', in which as well as transmitting information in a clear and accessible way, scientists are also listening and learning from laypeople's 'views, values, experiences, and concerns' (ibid.).

Trust in scientific research may be fragile, and it is vital that public engagement and consultation on extending the time limit for embryo research should be 'open, transparent, informed by evidence and should engage with the broad range

A modest extension of the limit might alternatively be justified by evidence that – very rarely – a single embryo can become conjoined twins *after* the primitive streak has formed, up to around 21 days (Blackshaw and Rodger 2021).

More permissively, it could be argued that – in a mirror image of the definition of death as brain stem death – the point at which the embryo's brain starts to develop (around 5 weeks) could represent the point after which it becomes unethical to carry out research on embryos. Sentience has also been argued to be 'a more defensible basis for embryo protection' than 'an appeal to individuation and neural development' (Castelyn 2020), and even if the capacity for sentience is defined extremely cautiously, this would allow for a significant extension to the 14 day limit. A further option would be to distinguish between different types of research, so that observational research is allowed beyond 14 days, while interventional research is not (Montgomery 2017). We could also adopt what lawyers refer to as 'backwards' reasoning to argue that, at 28 days, alternative sources of embryos become available, and hence placing the limit at 28 days is all that is needed.

The Risks of Reopening the 14 Day Limit

Much discussion of whether the 14 day limit should be changed appears to assume that any change would involve an extension of the time during which embryo research is permissible. It sometimes seems to be taken for granted that, if the public accepted the 14 day limit in 1990, then evidence that more valuable research could be carried out if the limit were extended would be likely to lead to public acceptance of a longer time limit. But while it might be hoped that extensive public engagement would indicate broad acceptance of the need for embryo research to continue, in addition to seeking agreement to an extension to the time limit, this is certainly not a foregone conclusion.

There are those – including Mary Warnock herself – who have cautioned against complacency when it comes to opening up the Human Fertilisation and Embryology Act 1990 for revision (Devolder 2017). Trust and distrust in scientists can be manipulated by the deliberate propagation of misinformation, and the so-called Pro-Life lobby is exceptionally well-organised and well-funded. Mary Warnock (2017) was concerned that reopening the 14 day limit might put the whole field of embryo research at risk, so that 'all the progress we have made since 1990 would be lost':

> pro-life people … are waiting in the wings and marshalling their forces to make an assault on what they regard as immoral legislation all over again. They will say: 'We always knew that the slippery slope would prove itself, and here it is, just as we said.' This is the reason why I want the 14-day rule to remain in place, at least for the time being. Perhaps with the 14-day rule we erred on the side of caution. But you cannot successfully block a slippery slope except by a fixed and invariable obstacle, which is what the 14-day rule provided.

It is likely that the overturning of *Roe v Wade* in 2022 will have given so-called Pro-Life campaigners renewed impetus to challenge long-standing liberal and permissive laws. If abortion can be banned in the US, after almost 50 years as a constitutional right, banning embryo research may seem eminently achievable.

Embryo Models

As we have seen, what are now called stem cell-based embryo models (SCBEMs) raise important new questions for the 14 day limit and the regulation of embryo research more generally. Under the Human Fertilisation and Embryology Act 1990, as amended, it is only lawful to carry out research on embryos if the research could not be done without using embryos. In addition to being necessary or desirable for one of the statutory purposes, the use of embryos in research must also be necessary. This 'necessity principle' requires the Licence Committee to reject an application for a research licence if there would be another way to carry out the research, for example, by using animal models, or human stem cell lines which have been deposited in the stem cell bank. If the research project could be carried out using SCBEMs instead of embryos, then the necessity principle would not be satisfied. Hence, the legislation creates an in-built presumption that – if SCBEMs could replace human embryos for research purposes – these models should be used in preference to human embryos.

It would, however, be a mistake to assume that SCBEMs will obviate the need for research on embryos. Most scientists accept that both will continue to be necessary. To take an obvious example, in order to validate the use of SCBEMs in research, it will be necessary to compare their development with human embryos.

This leads to the question of whether SCBEMs are, or should be subject to regulation in the same way as embryos, or are they merely engineered tissues that do not require special treatment, other than that which exists for research on other tissue samples? SCBEMs would only be subject to regulation by the HFEA if they were to qualify as 'embryos' for the purposes of the Human Fertilisation and Embryology Act 1990. As we saw earlier, section 1(1) of the Act sets out the meaning of 'embryo' for the purposes of the Act:

(1) In this Act (except in section 4A or in the term 'human admixed embryo') –

  (a) embryo means a live human embryo and does not include a human admixed embryo (as defined by section 4A(6)), and
  (b) references to an embryo include an egg that is in the process of fertilisation or is undergoing any other process capable of resulting in an embryo.

This is, as discussed earlier, an odd 'definition', since it contains the word it is supposed to be defining (an embryo means a … embryo). A better interpretation, and one endorsed by the House of Lords in *R (on the application of Quintavalle) v Secretary of State for Health* (2003) is that 'embryo' has its ordinary language meaning, and section 1(1) is instead specifying which *types* of embryo are covered by regulation. If the word 'embryo' is to be given its ordinary language meaning, then, on the one hand, a stem cell based embryo model is not an 'unborn human offspring', as per the Oxford English Dictionary. On the other hand, in *Quintavalle*, the House of Lords decided that CNR 'embryos' were embryos by 'construing new techniques in a way that incorporates them into the special regulatory framework' (Montgomery 2017). As we have seen, an overriding purpose of the Act was that there was to be 'no free for all' (*Quintavalle*, at [13]). Lord Steyn further explained that:

> Parliament intended the protective regulatory system in connection with human embryos to be comprehensive. This protective purpose was plainly not intended to be tied to the particular way in which an embryo might be created. The overriding ethical case for protection was general.
>
> (*Quintavalle*, at [26])

In terms of the application of the 'necessity principle', this leads to a conundrum. On the one hand, the 'necessity principle' in the Act would require SCBEMs to be used instead of human embryos whenever possible. On the other hand, SCBEMs will only be subject to regulation if they are categorised as embryos, in which case there is no longer a presumption that they should be used in preference to donated embryos. New rules are therefore necessary to clarify whether SCBEMs are embryos, for the purposes of the Act, and what limits should apply to their use. It will also be important for Parliament to decide whether the 'necessity principle' is still fit for purpose, and whether there even should be a presumption in favour of using SCBEMS, in preference to donated human embryos. It could, for example, plausibly be argued that the 'necessity principle' applies awkwardly here, since it might appear to suggest that allowing leftover embryos to perish is morally preferable to enabling patients to donate them for use in potentially valuable scientific research.

The difficulty of categorising new types of entity is not confined to embryo models. Classification difficulties also exist in relation to human-animal chimeras, and brain organoids, which in the future may 'manifest an ability to experience basic sensations such as pain, therefore manifesting sentience, or even rudimentary forms of consciousness' (Lavazza 2020). As Koplin and Gyngell (2020) put it, '[s]cientific advances are not only creating beings that blur or skirt existing categories; they are also calling these traditional categories into question'. This means that any revision of the 14 day limit might have to be accompanied by a clearer set of rules about what novel entities are covered by what regulation, as well as building in the possibility of future-proofing the regulatory scheme in order to accommodate entities which have not yet been produced or discovered.

Human embryo models also vary. Some non-integrated models 'mimic only specific aspects/tissues of human embryo development' (Clark et al. 2021), such as gastrulation. According to the ISSCR, these non-integrated models should be reported as part of an oversight process, but not normally subject to further review. In contrast, integrated embryo models which 'might realistically manifest the ability to undergo further integrated development if cultured for additional time in vitro should be subjected to a full specialized review' (ibid.). To put it simply and bluntly, if they were to develop the necessary extra-embryonic tissues, integrated embryo models might theoretically have the potential to implant, while non-integrated embryo models never could.

Unlike human embryos, it would be possible to generate very large quantities of SCBEMs for research purposes. At present, 'human embryos begin to degenerate as they approach the 14-day limit'. Despite progress in keeping embryos alive, Martin Pera has explained that 'only a minority will survive in a dish … and the number that remain healthy will diminish as development proceeds' (quoted in Servick 2021). Replacing human embryos with SCBEMs may enable different sorts of research to be carried out at scale, in a way that is impossible with the comparatively small number of donated embryos.

Currently, it is not entirely clear whether – if an embryo-like structure were to develop so that the primitive streak appeared – it would be legitimate to continue the research. If it is not an embryo, then it is not covered by regulation, and it could be allowed to develop with no time limit at all. But if it is sufficiently *like* an embryo that it has developed a primitive streak, should the legislation be interpreted expansively in order to ensure that there is no 'free for all'? If the decision was taken to err on the side of caution and include integrated embryo models within regulation, how does the 14 day limit apply to them? In practice, 'a new approach to regulation' may be required, not only because 'these entities would already have had an extended period in culture as stem cells' (Lovell-Badge et al. 2021), but also 'there is no "day zero" from which to begin counting' (Chan 2018). Embryo-like structures 'do not progress linearly; instead they mimic specific developmental points' (Matthews and Moralí 2020). This means that an embryo-like structure might mimic gastrulation earlier than 14 days, without the appearance of the primitive streak. Rather than using a time limit, it would instead be necessary to set limits based upon the structure of the entity and its capacity for development (Matthews and Moralí 2020).

According to the ISSCR guidelines, regulation should be extended to 'organized embryo-like cellular structure[s] with human organismal potential'. There are, however, difficulties in relying upon 'potential' as the defining feature which triggers regulation. First, if SCBEMs are subject to regulation only if they are capable of developing like a normal embryo, the experiments which would be necessary to establish this fact – through prolonged development *in vitro* or implantation in a woman's uterus – would themselves raise serious ethical issues (Rivron et al. 2018).

Secondly, before the discovery of somatic cell nuclear transfer and other ground-breaking developments, as Monika Piotrowska has pointed out, the definition of an embryo looked backwards, using fertilisation as the defining feature of an embryo (Piotrowska 2020). Once it became clear that 'embryos' could be created without fertilisation, that human embryonic stem cells might have the ability to develop into an organism (Thomson et al. 1998), and that human induced pluripotent stem cells could be reprogrammed to behave like embryonic stem cells (Takahashi 2007), new definitions were needed, and 'the new approach is to ignore the varied origins of cellular material and focus instead on the potential trajectory of some cells to grow into human beings' (Piotrowska 2020). But if many different types of cells could have potential, given the right environment, this sort of definition becomes over-inclusive. Piotrowska advocates instead concentrating upon 'morally salient facts' about an entity, such as 'the appearance of neural substrates and the functionality required for the experience of pain'.

If an embryo-like structure could be generated in a way that it did not develop a primitive streak, would that be a different way of avoiding the problem? As Rivron et al. (2018) explain:

> researchers might be able to constrain or enhance the developmental capacity of a particular model using gene editing – such as by incorporating suicide genes that destroy the tissue at a certain point. In other words, what might be considered an embryo could be flipped by genetic means into a non-embryo, and vice versa.

Chan notes a suggestion that embryo models could be produced in such a way that they lack full developmental potential, in order to ensure that research on them is legitimate, which she describes as an attempt 'to render embryos somehow "un-embryo" as a way of solving the moral problems associated with their use' (Chan 2018).

More complex questions still will arise if it ever becomes safe enough to use SCBEMs in treatment. It seems more likely that scientists will be able to create stem-cell derived sperm and eggs, which would then be used to create an embryo for use in treatment. This would have considerable advantages for people who are unable to use their own gametes in treatment, enabling them to have a child who was genetically 'theirs'. It is much less likely that anyone would ever contemplate the use of SCBEMs in treatment, especially since the 'embryo' would, in fact, be a clone of the tissue source. Laws are already in place in the UK which attempt to prevent 'rogue scientists' from attempting to do this, because under the Act no embryo other than a 'permitted embryo' can be used in treatment services. If, however, an SCBEM is not an embryo, there is no prohibition on its use. In any future law reform, a clear prohibition on the transplantation of embryo models into women's bodies is likely to serve as a 'red line' for the foreseeable future.

Notes

1 For example, Germany, Italy, Turkey, Russia and Austria (Matthews and Morali 2020).
2 By *Dobbs v. Jackson Women's Health Organization* (2022).
3 Early attempts to culture embryos for several days resulted in the embryo losing its integrity. Fishel et al. (1984) reported attempting to culture two embryos in vitro for 8–9 days. One expanded 'attaching to the surface of the petri dish between 189 and 216 hours post-fertilization. Its organization was lost as outgrowths, mostly trophoblastic', and the other 'became degenerate by 197 hours after insemination'.
4 It is, however, worth noting that making jewellery from a loved one's ashes or hair has become a growth industry, and is not viewed as disrespectful or contemptuous. British artist Helen Chadwick spent time as an artist-in-residence at King's College Hospital Assisted Conception Unit in 1995, where she produced jewellery and other images of the in vitro embryos.

5 The *Dobbs* (2022) decision in the US, which overturned *Roe v. Wade* (1973), is a salutary reminder not to take for granted access to reproductive healthcare. While only a small minority of parliamentarians are opposed to IVF in principle, they are likely to be vocal and well-organised in any future vote.
6 Analysis of discussions of the 14 day rule in Chinese social media found that 46.2% were neutral about an extension, 31.8% were supportive and 11.4% opposed extending the 14 day rule (Peng et al. 2022).

References

Appleby, John B. and Bredenoord, Annelien L. (2018) 'Should the 14-day rule for embryo research become the 28-day rule?' *EMBO Molecular Medicine* 10(9): e9437.

Blackshaw, Bruce Philip, and Rodger, Daniel (2021) 'Why we should not extend the 14-day rule' *Journal of Medical Ethics* 47(10): 712–714.

Callahan, D. (1995), 'The puzzle of profound respect' *Hastings Center Report* 25: 39–40.

Castelyn, Grant (2020) 'Embryo experimentation: is there a case for moving beyond the "14-day rule"' *Monash Bioethics Review* 38(2): 181–196.

Cavaliere, Giliua (2017) 'A 14-day limit for bioethics: the debate over human embryo research' *BMC Medical Ethics* 18(1): 1–12.

Chan, Sarah (2018) 'How and why to replace the 14-day rule' *Current Stem Cell Reports* 4(3): 228–234.

Chen, Chiann-Mun (Sheny) and Chisholm, Andrew (2017) 'Human development between 14 and 28 days' in *Human embryo culture: discussions concerning the statutory time limit for maintaining human embryos in culture in the light of some recent scientific developments* (Nuffield Council on Bioethics): 48–49.

Clark, Amander T et al. (2021) 'Human embryo research, stem cell-derived embryo models and *in vitro* gametogenesis: considerations leading to the revised ISSCR guidelines' *Stem Cell Reports* 16(6): 1416–1424.

Colomer, Modesto Ferrer and Pastor, Luis Miguel (2012) 'The preembryo's short lifetime: the history of a word' *Cuadernos de Bioética* 23(3): 677–694.

Cromer, Risa (2023) *Conceiving Christian America: embryo adoption and reproductive politics* (NYU Press).

Curran, Charles E. (1973) 'Abortion: law and morality in contemporary Catholic theology' *Jurist* 33: 162.

Devolder, Katrien (2017) 'The statutory time limit for maintaining human embryos in culture' in *Human embryo culture: discussions concerning the statutory time limit for maintaining human embryos in culture in the light of some recent scientific developments* (Nuffield Council on Bioethics): 78–80.

Diamond, James J. (1975) 'Abortion, animation, and biological hominization' (1975) *Theological Studies* 36(2): 305–324.

Elves, Charlotte and McGuinness, Sheelagh (2017) 'The statutory time limit for maintaining human embryos in culture' in *Human embryo culture: discussions concerning the statutory time limit for maintaining human embryos in culture in the light of some recent scientific developments* (Nuffield Council on Bioethics): 13–25.

Ethics Advisory Board (1979) HEW support of research involving human in vitro fertilization and embryo transfer (US Government Printing Office).

Fishel, S. B., Edwards, R. G., and Evans, C. J. (1984) 'Human chorionic gonadotropin secreted by preimplantation embryos cultured in vitro' *Science* 223(4638): 816–818.

Ford, Mary (2009) 'Nothing and not nothing: law's ambivalent response to transformation and transgression at the beginning of life' in S. Smith and R. Deazley (eds), *The legal, medical and cultural regulation of the body: transformation and transgression* (Routledge): 21–46.

House of Commons (2004) *Human reproductive technologies and the law: fifth report of session 2004–05* (House of Commons Science and Technology Committee).

Hyun, Insoo, Wilkerson, Amy, Johnston, Josephine (2016) 'Embryology policy: revisit the 14-day rule' Nature 533(7602): 169–171.

Hyun, Insoo, Bredenoord, Annelien L., Briscoe, James, Klipstein, Sigal, and Tan, Tao (2021) 'Human embryo research beyond the primitive streak' *Science* 371(6533): 998–1000.

Harris, John (2016) 'It's time to extend the 14-day limit for embryo research' *The Guardian* (6 May).

ISSCR (2021) 'Guidelines for stem cell research and clinical translation' retrieved from www.isscr.org/policy/guidelines-for-stem-cell-research-and-clinical-translation.

Jasanoff, Sheila (2011) 'Making the facts of life' in Sheila Jasanoff (ed.) *Reframing rights: bioconstitutionalism in the genetic age* (MIT Press): 59–85.

Johnston, Josephine, Baylis, Françoise and Greely, Henry T. (2021) 'ISSCR: grave omission of age limit for embryo research' *Nature* 594(7864): 495–495.

Koplin, Julian J. and Gyngell, Christopher (2020) 'Emerging moral status issues' *Monash Bioethics Review* 38(2): 95–104.

Lavazza, A. (2020) 'Human cerebral organoids and consciousness: a double-edged sword' *Monash Bioethics Review* 38(2): 105–128.

Lockwood, Michael (1988) 'Warnock versus Powell (and Harradine): when does potentiality count?' *Bioethics* 2(3): 187–213.

Lovell-Badge, Robin et al. (2021) 'ISSCR guidelines for stem cell research and clinical translation: the 2021 update' *Stem Cell Reports* 16(6): 1398–1408.

Ma, H. et al. (2019) '*In vitro* culture of cynomolgus monkey embryos beyond early gastrulation' *Science* 366(6467): p.eaax7890.

Matthews, Kirstin R.W. and Moralí, Daniel (2020) 'National human embryo and embryoid research policies: a survey of 22 top research-intensive countries' *Regenerative Medicine* 15(7): 1905–1917.

McCully, Sophia (2021) 'The time has come to extend the 14-day limit' *Journal of Medical Ethics* 47(12): e66.

McLaren, Anne (1984) 'Where to draw the line'. *Proceedings of the Royal Institute of Great Britain* 56: 101–121.

McLaren, Anne (1990) 'Research on the human conceptus and its regulation in Britain today' *Journal of the Royal Society of Medicine* 83(4): 209–213.

McMillan, Catriona (2021) 'When is human? Rethinking the fourteen-day rule' in Graeme Laurie et al. (eds) *The Cambridge handbook of health research regulation* (Cambridge University Press): 365–372.

Montgomery, Jonathan (2017) 'Introduction' in *Human embryo culture: discussions concerning the statutory time limit for maintaining human embryos in culture in the light of some recent scientific developments* (Nuffield Council on Bioethics): 3–11.

Moris, Naomi, Alev, Cantas, Pera, Martin and Martinez Arias, Alfonso (2021) 'Biomedical and societal impacts of *in vitro* embryo models of mammalian development' *Stem Cell Reports* 16(5): 1021–1030.

NIH Ad Hoc Group of Consultants to the Advisory Committee to the Director (1994) Report of the Human Embryo Research Panel (US Government Printing Office).

O'Donovan, Katherine (2006) 'Taking a neutral stance on the legal protection of the fetus' *Medical Law Review* 14(1): 115–123.

Peng, Y et al. (2022) 'A framework for the responsible reform of the 14-day rule in human embryo research' *Protein Cell* 13(8): 552–558.

Peters, Ted (2021) 'Keep the 14-day rule in stem cell research' *Theology and Science* 19(3): 177–183.

Piotrowska, Monika (2020) 'Avoiding the potentiality trap: thinking about the moral status of synthetic embryos' *Monash Bioethics Review* 38: 166–180.

Progress Educational Trust (2022) *Fertility, genomics and embryo research: public attitudes and understanding* (Progress Educational Trust).

Regaldo, Antonio (2021) 'Scientists plan to drop the 14 day rule, a key limit in stem cell research' *MIT Technology Review* (16 March).

Reincke, Cathelijne M., Bredenoord, Annelien L. and van Mil, Marc H.W. (2020) 'From deficit to dialogue in science communication: the dialogue communication model requires additional roles from scientists' *EMBO Reports* 21(9): e51278.

Rivron, Nicolas et al. (2018) 'Debate ethics of embryo models from stem cells' *Nature* 564(7735): 183–185.

Sawai, Tsutomu et al. (2020) 'The moral status of human embryo-like structures: potentiality matters? The moral status of human synthetic embryos' *EMBO Reports* 21(8): e50984.

Sawai, Tsutomu, Okui, Go, Akatsuka, Kyoko and Minakawa, Tomohiro (2021) 'Promises and rules: The implications of rethinking the 14-day rule for research on human embryos' *EMBO Reports* 22(9): e53726.

Servick, Kelly (2021) 'Door opened to more permissive research on human embryos' *Science* 372(6545): 894.

Steinbock, Bonnie (2007) 'The science, policy, and ethics of stem cell research' *Reproductive BioMedicine Online* 14(1): 130–136.

Subbaraman, Nidhi (2021) 'Limit on lab-grown human embryos dropped by stem-cell body' *Nature* 594: 18–19.

Suter, Sonia M. (2021) 'Legal challenges in reproductive genetics' *Fertility and Sterility* 115(2): 282.

Suter, Sonia M. (2022) 'Eroding lines in embryo research and abortion: contradictory slippery slopes' *Houston Journal of Health Law & Policy* 22: 7–51.

Takahashi, K. et al. (2007) 'Induction of pluripotent stem cells form adult human fibroblasts by defined factors' *Cell* 131(5): 861–872.

Thomson, J.A. et al. (1998) 'Embryonic stem cell lines derived from human blastocysts' *Science* 282(5391): 1145–1147.

Warnock, Mary (1985a) 'Moral thinking and government policy: the Warnock Committee on Human Embryology' *The Milbank Memorial Fund Quarterly: Health and Society* 63: 504–522.

Warnock, Mary (1985b) 'St Catherine's College seminars: the Warnock Report' *British Medical Journal* 291(6489): 187.

Warnock, Mary (2004) *Nature and mortality: recollections of a philosopher in public life* (Bloomsbury).

Warnock, Mary (2007) 'The ethical regulation of science' *Nature* 450(7170): 615.

Warnock, Mary (2017) 'Should the 14-day limit on human embryo research be extended' *Bionews* 9 (January).

Warnock Committee (1984) *Report of the Committee of Enquiry into Human Fertilisation and Embryology* (HMSO).

Williams, Kate, and Johnson, Martin H (2020) 'Adapting the 14-day rule for embryo research to encompass evolving technologies' *Reproductive Biomedicine & Society Online* 10: 1–9.

Wilson, Duncan (2011) 'Creating the "ethics industry": Mary Warnock, *in vitro* fertilization and the history of bioethics in Britain' *BioSocieties* 6: 121–141.

Zernicka-Goetz, Magdalena (2017) 'A need to expand our knowledge of early development' in *Human embryo culture: discussions concerning the statutory time limit for maintaining human embryos in culture in the light of some recent scientific developments* (Nuffield Council on Bioethics): 50–55.

Legal Judgments

St George's Healthcare NHS Trust v S [1998] All ER 673.
R (on the application of Quintavalle) v Secretary of State for Health [2003] 2 WLR 692.
Roe v. Wade 410 U.S. 113 (1973).
Dobbs v. Jackson Women's Health Organization, no. 19–1392 597 US (2022).

Parliamentary Debates

HL Deb (5 December 2002) vol. 641 col. 1327.

7 Conclusion

Summary of Principles and Proposals

In this book we have traced the history of the 14 day limit, and drawn attention to the pivotal roles played by Mary Warnock and Anne McLaren in its formulation and adoption. We have looked at the scientific and legislative histories of the 14 day rule, emphasising how tightly intertwined these are, and why we need a sociology of biotranslational science as well as robust governance structures – or, indeed, *in order* to formulate what these will be. This point is reinforced as we examine the legislative career, or evolution, of the 14 day rule over time, and the importance of its first premise of trustworthiness, enabling its second most important role as a guarantor of the 'conditional permissiveness' that allows scientific benefits to continue to be realised, even as they steadily move forward through controversial terrain such as embryo modelling. Throughout we have pointed out all of the ways that the 14 day limit has social and moral significance beyond its statutory power as a bright red line in the governance of embryo research, arguing that it embodies an approach to scientific research grounded in a social contract based on exchange between scientists, the state and the public. In exchange for allowing controversial research to be permissible, it will be subject to the strictest legal and regulatory oversight and sanctions.

As we have also argued, the 14 day rule necessarily reflects, embodies and expresses several different forms of reasoning. It balances the risk of legislation appearing 'slippery', arbitrary or partisan against the risk of having no regulation at all. It achieves this balance by setting the concept of what is absolutely true or right or good against the more pragmatic measure of what is alright to enough people to serve as an acceptable and therefore workable basis for governance. To some this is an unacceptable compromise, but as we have also shown, the exceptional success of this model over time sets a high bar. This is especially strongly confirmed by the absence of any other comparable legislative framework for regulating 'human fertilisation and embryology' anywhere else in the world – even 40 years after the Warnock Report which formed the basis for existing legislation was published. Despite being rock solid, moreover, the Warnock model of 'strict but permissive' regulation has facilitated the steady incorporation of new and often controversial scientific developments since 1990, including cell nuclear replacement, stem cell research and human admixed embryos. The question society now faces is how this long-established model of 'strict but permissive' regulation should apply to calls

DOI: 10.4324/9781003294108-7

for the extension of the 14 day limit, given its role as a cornerstone of such a popular and uniquely successful regulatory framework, and to the challenges posed for regulation by embryo models.

Looking ahead, we should remember that the 14 day limit was not only a compromise solution to implacable and irresolvable disagreement about whether it could ever be legitimate to carry out research on human embryos, but also something of an experiment. The Warnock Committee was never going to be able to come up with a blueprint for legislation which satisfied everyone, and, as we have seen, a minority of the Committee dissented on the question of embryo research. Legislation could never be capable of neutralising opposition to embryo research: there will always be people to whom it is an article of faith that the embryo is a person from the moment of conception. But the Warnock Consensus is not dependent upon universal agreement, rather it is based on establishing regulatory principles and mechanisms that are capable of providing *sufficient* reassurance to *enough* people to be acceptable. This ability to balance competing and/or opposing interests and positions, in the most accommodating manner, while still delivering firm guidelines is one of the most valuable lessons to be learned from the 14 day rule's now lengthy history.

Despite the existence of profound moral disagreement about the legitimacy of the instrumental use of human embryos, the 14 day rule – as a strict limit, which sets an absolute boundary for scientific research – has undoubtedly helped to foster public trust and confidence in research. This trust in turn has helped to propel forward a remarkably generous civic environment of participation in and support for translational bioscience in the UK. Another of the most important lessons to be learned from the 'virtuous circle' the 14 day rule has helped to promote is that rules are symbols and expressive emblems of social values – not just red lines that can't be crossed.

A sociological perspective helps to remind us too that the same principle of reciprocity that underlines the fundamental exchange in the social contract that allows controversial embryo research to be allowed subject to very strict conditions of oversight and regulation is also embedded in the NHS, and in scientific culture in the UK more generally. As we have seen, although it is often not an available option, IVF patients commonly express a preference for donating embryos to research. Overwhelmingly, such donations to research are described in the classically open-ended altruistic language of 'giving something back', by potentially improving outcomes for future patients (Kvernflaten et al. 2022), and it is interesting that this sort of 'public good' altruism is usually preferred to making a 'gift of life' to another infertile couple or person. Of course, this preference is by no means solely attributable to the strict limits on embryo research. Potential embryo donors may also be concerned that their donated embryo could result in the birth of a child who is a full genetic sibling of their own children, and who might contact them in the future. Nevertheless, a common preference for donation to research suggests that IVF patients in general have a high level of trust and confidence that there has been no 'free for all', and that research on embryos only takes place under strict regulation. Indeed, it could be argued that the legal and practical obstacles to donation – such as requiring donation to be a specific project of research – routinely thwart patient preferences, and that a move towards embryo banking, and broad consent, would be a better way of protecting patients' interests.

The legitimacy of research on embryos is not alone as an issue on which there could never be agreement within society. Abortion and assisted dying are also characterised by profound and immovable disagreement, often on moral grounds. While the 14 day limit has by no means extinguished opposition to embryo research, it is noteworthy that the 'heat' has largely been taken out of the issue, and – in comparison with abortion and assisted dying – there is relatively little ongoing debate over the morality of embryo research.

Indeed, it is worth noting that the UK's success in coming up with a comprehensive and strict-but-permissive regulatory scheme for embryo research stands in direct opposition to its failure to reform archaic abortion laws, under which abortion is still prima facie a criminal offence, unless two doctors agree that the pregnant woman's health would be more at risk from pregnancy than termination (Offences Against the Person Act 1861; Abortion Act 1967). In relation to assisted dying too, the UK is hardly a trailblazer of permissive regulation (Jackson 2022). We cannot therefore trace the UK's pioneering legislation on fertilisation and embryology to the UK Parliament's inherently liberal and permissive approach to questions that go to the value and meaning of human life.

If, as we would argue, the 14 day limit has been a remarkable success, what lessons might this have for policy makers in other settings? First, the extended deliberative process that led up to the Warnock Report was important. As Charis Thompson (2013) has put it, 'good science' depends upon 'satisfying public concerns', which in turn requires honest and clear communication and the building of trust:

> Good science cannot be achieved or legislated once and for all. It is ongoing and iterative, and it requires openness to dissent and the best work of many different kinds of contributors.

The Warnock Committee had the time and the expertise, as well as the independence, to consider the issues in depth, and – tellingly – to produce a short and tightly focussed report. The Warnock Report, including the dissents and list of recommendations is only 94 pages long. In contrast, the recent report on surrogacy by the Law Commission of England and Wales and the Scottish Law Commission runs to 587 pages (Law Commissions 2023). Appointing a diverse group of skilled people, and giving them the resources they needed, was key to Warnock's success – but drafting by committee is also notoriously fraught with difficulty. As we have seen, Mary Warnock and Anne McLaren played a foundational role in the Committee's work and their style of leadership was highly effective. Their empathetic and compassionate attitude towards infertility, and their brisk, no-nonsense search for a compromise resulted in a set of clear and unambiguous recommendations that continue to form the bedrock of the regulation of fertility treatment and embryo research four decades later. Notably, the Warnock Committee recommendations were not enacted for seven years after they were drafted, and huge credit for the shift in hearts and minds that led to the establishment of the Human Fertilisation and Embryology Authority in 1991 belongs with the members of the scientific and medical communities who worked tirelessly alongside sympathetic parliamentarians and government ministers to achieve this outcome.

Duncan Wilson, in his history of British bioethics, has drawn attention to the fact that the choice of Mary Warnock as the Committee's chair 'came amidst, and reflected, growing calls for external oversight of science and medicine', and that she then 'used her position as chair to publicly endorse greater oversight of science and medicine' (Wilson 2011). But what Warnock and McLaren foresaw is that this external oversight and control was to the *benefit* of researchers, by conferring legitimacy on their work, and proving that 'knowledge can be pursued without being put to morally intolerable uses' (Warnock 1988). McLaren in particular had great faith in the ability of the general public to appreciate the obvious benefits of IVF and embryo research – a prediction that has been hugely confirmed by the rapid normalisation of IVF over the past three decades.

In her own commentary on the Warnock Report, Mary Warnock (1985) was clear that everyone had a right to make their own decisions in 'matters of life and death, of birth and the family':

> For these are areas that are central to morality, and everyone has a right to judge for himself. Such issues indeed lie at the heart of society; everyone not only wants to make their own choices but are bound to do so. And this is why there cannot be moral experts. Everyone's choice is his own.

Both our emphasis on the importance of 'conditional permissiveness' and of 'beneficial limits' reflect our appreciation of the need to balance respect for the diversity of public opinion on controversial matters of life and death with the need to provide clear guidelines for scientific research in fields such as human embryo research. As the 14 day rule demonstrates, it is possible to both accommodate diametrically opposing views and to provide a clear way forward for science if the regulatory infrastructure is built on principles of compromise, such as the Warnockian view that legislation does not need to be 'right' for everyone in order to be 'right enough' for a sufficient majority to enable some legislation to take the place of none. Similarly, it is helpful to acknowledge, as Warnock often did, that limits are not necessarily weakened by being somewhat arbitrary. Indeed many laws are somewhat arbitrary, and it neither follows that they are entirely so, nor that it is necessarily problematic if they are changed. Both of these principles reflect the passionate belief shared by Warnock and McLaren that good science can be protected through progressive legislation, and that the public will have greater trust in science when they perceive it is subject to credible enforcement and oversight.

In short, reproduction matters, and the research on human embryos which made IVF possible has transformed the IVF platform into one of the most successful translational technologies of the twentieth century. This process of biotranslation – from basic science to whole new fields of clinical application and in turn to yet other new avenues of biological discovery – has also shown how much the process of successful translation relies on public engagement, robust legislation, the active role of government, well-administered and respected regulators and strong support from professional bodies. It also demonstrates the multifaceted nature of the complex biotranslational process, and why a sociological perspective is a key element in understanding this complexity.

Progressive Legislation in the 1980s

A central claim in this book has been that the 14 day limit has played a key role in facilitating the translational success of IVF, and that this is part of the much larger sociological picture we should keep in mind as we assess the question of what kind of regulatory infrastructure needs to evolve from here in order to take into account not only of new reproductive, but also new regenerative possibilities. With the benefit of hindsight, what we now know is that the 14 day rule provided an extraordinarily successful regulatory solution to the difficult problem of what to do about a controversial new scientific development (successful human IVF) in the face of intractable disagreements over its moral legitimacy, a legal vacuum and a suspicious public. Without the secure grounding the 14 day rule and its accompanying logics provided for the comprehensive legislative architecture built around them, IVF would likely have become highly restricted in the UK and this would undoubtedly have had a huge effect worldwide. Instead, the opposite sequence of events unfolded: IVF and embryo research became the centrepiece and fulcrum of a broad argument about the promise of scientific research, and the crucial role of regulation in enabling and protecting it. This protection in turn solidified yet another crucial union – between good regulation and good science. As the 14 day rule became both an enabler and an emblem of this translational path forward, it became a flagship global standard for not only the fertility industry but all the myriad spin offs from the IVF and embryo transfer platform – from transgenic sheep farms to egg freezing clinics. In turn, this legacy of strict-but-permissive regulation has now ushered in a new era in which reproductive and regenerative research increasingly overlap – a conjunction embodied in the new science of embryo modelling.

This entire sequence of events was never a foregone conclusion. That the UK was able to enact the first comprehensive and permissive system for the regulation of human fertilisation and embryology under a Conservative government, led by a Prime Minister who had herself espoused a return to 'Victorian values' (Samuel 1992), is truly remarkable, and suggests that it is worth paying close attention to what made this possible. Margaret Thatcher's government's approach to matters of human reproduction was hardly liberal and inclusive. Introducing what would become known as Section 28 of the Local Government Act 1988 – which prohibited schoolteachers from promoting homosexuality or its acceptability 'as a pretended family relationship' – Margaret Thatcher bemoaned the fact that 'children who need to be taught to respect traditional moral values are being taught that they have the inalienable right to be gay' (Thomas 1993).

Of course, the factors behind the eventual passage of the Human Fertilisation and Embryology Act are many and varied, and beyond the scope of this book, but it is our contention that the 14 day rule played an important role in sidestepping irresolvable moral disagreements, and instead focussing on devising a workable set of limits that could be readily understood and strictly enforced, in order to promote public confidence and trust.

Principles and Proposals

The interrelated and overlapping principles which underlie the Warnock approach to regulation, embodied by the 14 day rule, can be simply stated. The first is that strict regulation can be a facilitator of science, rather than a hindrance or an obstruction to it. Secondly, clear, principled and agreed upon limits are an effective means to respond to public concern in response to controversial scientific developments. Being prepared to draw strict red lines, and ensure a persuasive means of enforcing them, helps to promote and engender public trust. Thirdly, and crucially, public concern about novel scientific developments is a crucial resource to be drawn upon in the process of devising effective legislation, not something to be seen as a hindrance or impediment to science. As the UK has learned through both positive and negative experience, taking public concerns seriously is an essential prerequisite for regulation that will itself be capable of facilitating scientific progress.

We have also argued that there are important lessons to be learned from the essentially reciprocal model of exchange that underlies the Warnock Consensus: that *in exchange* for allowing IVF and embryo research to be permitted they will be subject to the very strictest oversight and regulation, including the use of criminal law. It is consistent with the gift model offered by Richard Titmuss that a reciprocal social contract of this kind engenders greater public trust. The now widespread evidence of more support than opposition among the public for the use of embryos in research supports Titmuss's view that reciprocity and trust are closely related, perhaps especially in relation to healthcare. As mentioned earlier, a YouGov survey from 2017 found considerable public support for extending the 14 day limit, and this finding has since been confirmed in several other studies. In 2022, the Progress Educational Trust (PET) commissioned IPSOS to carry out a public opinion survey (involving a representative sample of 2233 UK adults) of attitudes towards fertility, genomics and embryo research. It found that twice as many supported research on embryos, compared with those who opposed it. People who answered this question were also asked about the 14 day rule. Was it too long, too short or about right? By far the largest percentage – 56 per cent – thought it was about right, while 9 per cent said it was too long and 13 per cent thought it was too short. A second supplementary question exploring what type of research might justify extending the limit to 28 days revealed the highest levels of support for research aimed at finding new treatments for congenital diseases (39 per cent), improving medical understanding of stillbirth (35 per cent) and improving medical understanding of miscarriage (33 per cent). Still more recently, in 2023, the HDBI public consultation on the 14 day rule similarly found that a significant majority the public were in favour of extending it – a finding which, as noted earlier, many respondents favouring extension linked specifically to the goal of improving the success IVF treatment.

As this book goes to press, the Wellcome-funded Human Developmental Biology Initiative and UKRI Sciencewise are together engaging in an extensive programme of public dialogue workshops,[1] a key purpose of which is to 'Use this initial evidence base to inform future public engagement, policy decisions and reviews around regulations governing research on human embryos, such as the 14-day rule.'

At the same time, Cambridge Reproduction has launched the Governance of Stem Cell-Based Embryo Models (G-SCBEM) project, bringing together scientists, lawyers, bioethicists funders and regulators, and consulting widely, in order to produce 'a clear and comprehensive recommended governance framework for research using SCBEMs' (University of Cambridge 2023). The intention is to devise interim voluntary, consensual and robust governance principles in consultation with other national and international oversight bodies in order to inform and accelerate the crucial process of filling the legal void that currently surrounds the use of embryo models.

Embryo models pose a critical stress test for the current UK statutory system both because they lie outside its remit and because they pose new types of ethical, legal and social questions related to embryo research. Given that work on them is not only underway, but developing quickly, there is some degree of urgency to solving the question of how they are and should be regulated. Should they be subject to exactly the same regulatory scheme as existing research embryos, or is a different approach required? Should a distinction be drawn between integrated embryo models which closely mimic natural embryological development, and non-integrated models which do not? Is the HFEA the right regulator for all types of embryo research, or might it be more sensible to draw up a memorandum of understanding between the Human Tissue Authority, the Medical Research Council, the Stem Cell Bank and the HFEA? Is a licensing regime, backed up by criminal sanctions, a proportionate way to regulate embryo models?

In trying to work out what limits should be placed on the use of embryo models in research, it might be important to consider whether they share with embryos some sort of 'special' moral status? Should there, for example, be limits on the purposes for which research can be carried out on embryo models? It is possible rapidly to manufacture hundreds of thousands of embryo models, so does this alter the current requirement that research should be carried out only for specific purposes? Would it, for example, be acceptable or even sensible to use them in toxicology testing to identify whether medicines taken by pregnant women are likely to have teratogenic effects? Would it be preferable to replace the current list of defined statutory purposes with a 'public good' requirement? Are there fresh considerations, such as the provenance of stem cells, which need to be part of the regulatory regime?

A key question is what limit should apply to embryo models, which have the potential to add significantly to knowledge which might illuminate the 14 to 28 day period – or beyond. Such knowledge could offer important insights into the origins of congenital disease as well as the causes of miscarriages and stillbirths. The 14 to 28 day period might also be of particular importance in understanding the causes of IVF's high failure rate. As noted above, these are all areas the public would like to see prioritised if post-14 day embryo modelling is allowed to proceed subject to regulation. The 2021 ISSCR guidelines suggest that integrated embryo models should be cultivated 'for the minimum time necessary to achieve the scientific objective' (para. 2.2.2g) but this is a fairly flexible definition.

The ISSCR has also strongly recommended more research into public perceptions of both embryo modelling and the question of extending the 14 day rule. They have also urged government to engage more fully and purposefully with the statutory challenge posed by embryo-like entities which could, in theory, become viable embryos that have the equivalent developmental potential to embryos produced through fertilisation. Given the UK's prominent role in leading both research and policy in the field of human fertilisation and embryology, there is a logic to exploring a UK-based, voluntary regulatory system that could serve as a template, or even default set of oversight guidelines and limits for other countries. Such a UK-based system could include a Code of Practice outlining permissible uses of embryo models as well as impermissible activities such as the use of embryo models for reproductive purposes in humans – or in any mammals. Guidelines would also be likely to cover the sources of research materials, consent procedures, documentation of materials and methods and the storage, banking and transfer of embryo models. The voluntary implementation of a rigorous system of oversight by a dedicated Steering Committee linked to exiting research funders and regulators could be undertaken in exchange for extending the upper time limit on embryo research to 21 or 28 days.

A starting point for such a process might be a set of strictly prohibited activities informed by exactly the kind of public engagement that is currently underway, and also widespread consultation with both national and international regulators and professional scientific bodies such as the Royal Society, the European Society for Human Reproduction and Embryology, the HFEA, and the ISSCR. In previous cases of novel policy formation, including the formation of the HFEA, the Asilomar agreements related to recombinant DNA, and the worldwide ban on using gene editing for human reproductive purposes, voluntary systems of compliance and oversight have made important and substantial contributions to scientific governance. While there is understandable caution about letting the scientific community create its own rules, it is equally the case that important historical policy changes have started in exactly that manner.

New Model Legislation

As we consider these questions it may be wise to remember that embryo models are themselves the offspring not only of IVF, embryo research and remarkable new methods of *in vitro* culture of embryoids derived from a variety of cell-based and non-cell-based sources. They are also the offspring of the 14 day rule and the highly successful research culture this has helped to engender worldwide. A radical, but undoubtedly timely question to ask in the wake of the creation of embryo models is what kind of legal vacuum needs now to be filled, exactly. Clearly it is not the same one the 14 day rule ushered into legislative viability more than 30 years ago. The legal vacuum surrounding the embryo model is in many ways nothing like the complete absence of any governance procedures to oversee clinical IVF in the wake of the birth of the world's first test tube baby – now nearly half a century ago.

With this in mind, it is important to take a step back from the embryo model per se and ask what governance is for? Surely Mary Warnock was right when she claimed that the law is an expression of social morality, collectivity and obligation – not just regulation for the sake of having rules. And just as surely both she and Anne McLaren rightly judged that the underlying issue of the 'legal vacuum' was key to public confidence and trust. If, then, we begin not with the empty vessel of the legal vacuum, but the at-least-half-full glass of public trust, three key tasks await our deliberation, and most likely need to be investigated simultaneously.

The first of these has to be the acquisition of better knowledge about public perceptions of new reproductive and regenerative research projects more generally. This might yield some very important findings. For example, it might be that we discover it is not the science of fertility or embryo modelling people are worried about so much as the commercialism of the fertility industry, the high cost of fertility care, the uneven lottery of NHS-funded IVF provision, or the high failure rate of many IVF-based procedures. Recent research on egg freezing, for example, has shown that many women feel extremely disappointed and often angry in the wake of undergoing this procedure – and for reasons that would not have been obvious without careful research.[2] The general public may be more concerned about misuses of biological data, or the use of AI in IVF, than in either embryo models or gene editing. At the moment, we simply do not know.

A second question that needs to be asked is what the scientific community can already agree on in terms of prohibited, impermissible and unethical research in the area of human fertilisation and embryology– as well as what are the priority areas for research and why. The former is already a fairly long list including human cloning, the use of CRISPR for reproductive purposes,[3] the implantation of animal embryos in humans or vice versa and the use of human embryo models for clinical purposes. But there are many other agreed-upon principles and standards that have been developed over the past two decades in particular that would bear spelling out more explicitly. These include the very strict requirements related to the use of human cell-based technologies, in particular in terms of their labelling, characterisation, standardisation, storage, provenance and handling as well as storage. The consent procedures for donation of embryos to research are robust and elaborate. Ethical review processes are well-established, and most scientists take seriously their duties of openness and transparency. All of these issues are part of the same ecosystem that connects scientific research to people's lives, and scientific research to social values.

A third key point is the one mentioned earlier – that IVF has completely transformed both the clinical and the research landscape of 'human fertilisation and embryology' over the past half-century. This 'IVF-effect' has had a huge influence. The very fact that IVF is now so completely taken for granted is the ultimate translational test. Being 'after IVF' not only means it now such a well-known reproductive option it has essentially become routine. It also means that the role of technology in 'assisting' something so basic and intimate as human reproduction has also been normalised. If we have, in a sense, already turned the human embryo into means of better understanding our own biology, perhaps this is not only an important social and biological fact but also a significant moral as well as cultural and scientific turning point? Such a shift would mean that the ability of IVF to 'mimic' or replicate – or indeed to replace altogether – the process of human conception has become part of the cultural vernacular. It suggests that, like the famous NASA image of the blue earth, the horizon-like image of the micromanipulated embryo is now a shorthand for the future of assisted human biology. Surely if this is one way to describe the cultural implications of the 'IVF-ication' of human reproduction such a change in public perceptions has huge implications for what counts as a 'trustworthy' technology.

With all of these issues in mind, it may be that the 14 day rule has served its purpose and that no single time limit is appropriate for all scientific research involving human embryos – especially now that the category of embryo overlaps with the large and diverse group of entities deemed to be embryo-like. It may be that some forms of embryo research – for example exploratory embryo modelling – will need to be regulated in terms of purposes and uses, so that material used solely for research purposes is regulated differently from anything that might be used clinically. Such divisions are already part of the stem cell therapy landscape, and they may be more relevant than the 14 day rule (or even the 21 or 28 day rule) to embryo modelling, embryoid-ology and the inevitable successor projects of the human embryome and embryomics.

Three things we know for sure are that good regulation is not just about prohibition, limits and bright lines. Good regulation protects research as well as the public, and enables progressive adaptations so long as they are aligned with basic principles of constraint, oversight and accountability. Another thing we know is that although people want 'some limit rather than none', they are also aware that limits can – and should – be changed over time. The reasons people want some limits rather than none are the important point to keep in focus, because ultimately what people do not want is governance they do not trust. A third certainty is that whatever regulatory mechanisms evolve in the future they will do so iteratively – in a step-by-step process that will vary country to country and in response to continuously changing scientific understandings of human reproduction and development. With these points in mind, we should be confident that drafting successful regulation for human fertilisation and embryology in the future is not only feasible and already starting to take shape, but that we have a very impressive legacy to build upon.

Notes

1 See further https://hdbi.org/public-engagement.
2 Greenwood et al. (2018) found that nearly half of all women who had frozen their eggs experienced some 'decision regret'. Relevant factors included the degree of support women received during the procedure and the adequacy of the information they received. For example, six per cent of women believed that their probability of achieving a live birth with frozen eggs was 100 per cent, and unrealistic expectations of success increased

the chance of experiencing regret. As well as accurate information about success rates, it is important that women are given information about how many women return to use their frozen eggs, in Kakkar et al.'s study (2023), only 16 per cent had done so.

3 Jiankui's unethical use of CRISPR led to worldwide condemnation, but it is not clear that the risks of using CRISPR in fertility treatment will continue to outweigh the risks indefinitely (Kirksey 2023).

References

Greenwood, Eleni A., Pasch, Lauri A. Hastie, Jordan, Cedars, Marcelle I. and Huddleston, Heather G. (2018) 'To freeze or not to freeze: decision regret and satisfaction following elective oocyte cryopreservation' *Fertility and sterility* 109: 1097–1104.

Jackson, Emily (2022) *Medical law*, 6th edition (Oxford University Press): ch. 17.

Kakkar, Pragati et al. (2023) 'Outcomes of social egg freezing: a cohort study and a comprehensive literature review' *Journal of Clinical Medicine* 12: 4182.

Kirksey, Eben (2023) 'Does gene editing have a future in reproductive medicine?' *New York Times* (4 March).

Kvernflaten, B., Fedorcsák, P. and Solbrække, K.N. (2022) 'Kin or research material? Exploring IVF couples' perceptions about the human embryo and implications for disposition decisions in Norway' *Bioethical Inquiry* 19, 4: 571–585.

Law Commissions (2023) *Building families through surrogacy: a new law*, Law Com no. 411, Scottish Law Com no. 262 (Law Commission of England and Wales and Scottish Law Commission).

McLaren, Anne (2004) 'A conversation with Dr Anne McLaren, DBE, DPhil, FRS, FRCOG' *Human Fertility* 7(2): 83–89.

Progress Educational Trust (2022) *Fertility, genomics and embryo research: public attitudes and understanding* (Progress Educational Trust 2022).

Samuel, Raphael (1992) 'Mrs. Thatcher's return to Victorian values' *Proceedings of the British Academy* 78: 9–29.

Thomas, Philip A. (1993) 'The nuclear family, ideology and AIDS in the Thatcher years' *Feminist Legal Studies* 1: 23.

Thompson, Charis. (2013) *Good science: the ethical choreography of stem cell research* (MIT Press).

University of Cambridge (2023) 'Project launched to provide guidance on research using human stem cell-based embryo models' retrieved from www.cam.ac.uk/research/news/project-launched-to-provide-guidance-on-research-using-human-stem-cell-based-embryo-models.

Warnock, Mary (1985) *A question of life: the Warnock Report on human fertilisation and embryology* (Basil Blackwell).

Warnock, Mary (1988) 'A national ethics committee' *British Medical Journal* 297: 1626–1627.

Wilson, Duncan (2011) 'Creating the "ethics industry": Mary Warnock, *in vitro* fertilization and the history of bioethics in Britain' *BioSocieties* 6: 121–141.

Index